ACCLAIM F

THE SHO

SA ⠀⠀⠀ RY

"Drs. Kaplowitz and Barc
about the causes of shor
endocrinologists evaluate ⸻
affect growth. The different therapies—including growth
hormones—that are available for the short child are
presented in an easy-to-understand way, along with
realistic expectations about responses to therapy."

—Scott A. Rivkees, MD, professor of pediatric endocrinology,
director, Yale Child Health Research Center,
Yale University School of Medicine

"Accurate, easily understood, and to-the-point [regarding] parents' most frequently asked questions, THE SHORT CHILD is the only reference that speaks directly to parents of children with short stature. Today, human growth hormones are a controversial topic, and the authors take a balanced approach to the issue."

—Alan D. Rogol, MD, PhD, professor of pediatrics,
University of Virginia

"Drs. Kaplowitz and Baron carefully review medical and social issues, present risks and benefits clearly and fairly, and make thoughtful recommendations."

—Leslie Plotnick, MD, professor of pediatrics,
Johns Hopkins Medical Institutions,
clinical director, Pediatric Endocrinology

more . . .

"A thorough depiction of what all parents should know and understand about their child's growth."

"Kaplowitz and Baron provide parents with an unusually comprehensive and accessible guide to the medical and psychological aspects of growth. THE SHORT CHILD offers sound and practical suggestions while emphasizing that the 'right' decision regarding treatment depends as much on the individual child and family as it does on the diagnosis."

THE
SHORT
CHILD

A Parents' Guide to the Causes,
Consequences, and Treatment
of Growth Problems

PAUL KAPLOWITZ, MD, PhD,
Chief of Endocrinology,
Children's National Medical Center
and
JEFFREY BARON, MD,
Pediatric Endocrinologist

**WARNER
WELLNESS**

NEW YORK   BOSTON

This book is not intended to function as a substitute for the medical advice of a treating physician or to encourage the diagnosis of any illness, disease, or medical problem by laypersons. Please consult with your child's doctor. The application of any recommendation set forth in this book is at the reader's discretion and risk.

The individuals and growth charts described in this book are designed to illustrate a concept and may not represent a single patient.

Copyright © 2006 by Jeffrey Baron, MD, and Paul Kaplowitz, MD, PhD
All rights reserved.

Warner Wellness, an imprint of Warner Books, Inc.

Hachette Book Group, USA
1271 Avenue of the Americas, New York, NY 10020

Warner Wellness and the Warner Wellness logo are trademarks of Time Inc. used under license.

Printed in the United States of America

First Edition: June 2006
10 9 8 7 6 5 4 3 2 1

Library of Congress Cataloging-in-Publication Data

Kaplowitz, Paul.
    The short child : a parents' guide to the causes, consequences, and treatment of growth problems / Paul Kaplowitz and Jeffrey Baron.—1st ed.
        p.   cm.
    Includes index.
    ISBN-13: 978-0-446-69652-4
    ISBN-10: 0-446-69652-8
    1. Children—Growth—Popular works.   2. Growth disorders—Popular works.   I. Baron, Jeffrey.   II. Title.

RJ131.K363   2006
618.92'4—dc22

                                            2005029231

Contents

You probably first became aware that your child was short when you saw him or her next to other children of the same age—cousins possibly, or friends, or perhaps other children in day care. Alternatively, you might have learned of the short stature during a visit to a pediatrician who weighed and measured and then told you that your child was "off the growth charts."

For many parents, the discovery that their child's height is below the normal range is confusing and distressing. As pediatric endocrinologists, we receive numerous phone calls and clinic visits from concerned parents with questions about short stature. *Why is my child short? Is there a medical problem? How tall will my child be as an adult? Should we be doing something about it? Is there a particular diet that helps growth?* Many parents know that the Food and Drug Administration (FDA) recently approved growth hormone to treat children who are very short for no known reason, and they wonder whether their child should be taking growth hormone. Even parents of children who are within the normal range but below average are often concerned that their child will be at a disadvantage socially, athletically, or professionally.

The Short Child is for parents who are seeking information, trying to understand why their child is short, whether there is an underlying medical problem, how they can optimize growth, and whether their child should be receiving medical treatment. It was written to provide straightforward answers to the many questions that parents have. The information provided is based on studies in the medical literature, tempered by our own experience as pediatric endocrinologists who have been evaluating and treating children with growth disorders for many years.

We'll begin by introducing the extraordinary process of growth that transforms a tiny embryo into an adult. We will explain the influence of genetics on height, providing a way for you to calculate the expected height of your children based on your own height and your spouse's. We include practical information about the essential role of nutrition in growth, explaining when you should be concerned about your child's nutrition and providing guidance about ways to improve nutrition if needed. We'll also explore the key hormones that regulate growth, focusing especially on growth hormone, and discuss the social and psychological effects of short stature and how parents can help their child maintain a positive outlook.

Your main question may be simply, *Is my child's height normal or abnormal?* We'll explain how growth specialists address this question, how growth charts are used to determine a child's height percentile and assess the overall pattern of growth, and how body weight, general health, and family heights all must be considered. Methods to predict adult height are discussed, and guidelines given to help you decide whether your child should be evaluated by a growth specialist.

We will discuss the many causes of short stature. Most short children are healthy, but there are some who grow poorly because of an underlying medical problem. We'll explain the tests that a physician will perform to sort out these causes.

We'll discuss medical approaches to treat children who are extremely short—including growth hormone, male hormones, and delay of puberty—and note how much or how little benefit these approaches can provide. These benefits must be weighed against the drawbacks of therapy, including the known side effects, the possible risks, and the costs, as well as the possible psychological risks of labeling the child's physical difference as a disease. There are also ethical and societal issues that make growth hormone treatment for short children with no known medical problem very controversial.

As pediatric endocrinologists, we have been listening to

parents and teaching them about growth for years. Often parents have so many questions, it is difficult to answer them all fully during a clinic or office visit. *The Short Child* was written to provide more comprehensive answers, to help allay excessive concern, and, when needed, to help parents interact with their child's doctor more knowledgeably to obtain the care that their child needs.

THE
SHORT
CHILD

CHAPTER 1

The Normal Pattern of Growth

WHAT CAUSES CHILDREN TO GROW?

Growth is a remarkable process that transforms a microscopic embryo into a newborn baby approximately 20 inches long, and eventually into an adult, usually between 5 and 6 feet tall. Biomedical research has provided great insights into human growth, although much remains to be learned. We know that children grow larger because the cells throughout their body enlarge and then divide to form two cells. Then each of those cells enlarges and divides again.

A child's height is primarily determined by the length of his or her bones, and thus children grow taller because their bones grow longer. The bones grow longer because they contain growth plates. These are thin layers of cartilage found near the ends of the bones. Cartilage is a firm, resilient material found in your ears and nose, as well as lining the ends of your bones at the joints. Children also have cartilage farther inside the bones, forming the growth plates (figure 1). Within the growth plates, cells divide and enlarge, producing more cartilage, which is subsequently converted into bone. This process causes the bones to elongate.

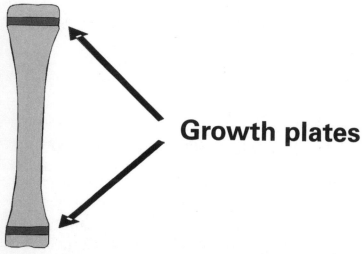

Growth plates

Figure 1. A diagram of a bone showing the positions of the growth plates. Vertebrae (the bones that form the spine) also have growth plates.

GROWTH IS RAPID EARLY IN LIFE, THEN SLOWS

Prior to birth, your child grew at an enormous rate, starting as a microscopic fertilized egg and then growing about 20 inches and about 6 to 9 pounds in the nine months of pregnancy. If that growth rate were to continue after birth, the child would reach adult size in two or three years! However, the growth rate slows down with age (see table 1). In the first year after birth, an average child grows about 10 inches in length. In the second year, a child usually grows about 5 inches. By the time he or she is seven years old, the average child is only growing about 2 inches per year.

Table 1. Typical Growth Rates at Different Ages

Age	Growth Rate
0–1 year (first year of life)	10 inches per year
1–2 years (second year of life)	5 inches per year
4–5 years	2½ inches per year
7–9 years	2¼ inches per year
Middle of adolescent growth spurt (boys)	3½ inches per year
Middle of adolescent growth spurt (girls)	3 inches per year

THE ADOLESCENT GROWTH SPURT

This progressive decline in the growth rate is interrupted by the adolescent growth spurt (also known as the pubertal growth spurt). Sometime after puberty starts, the child's growth speeds up for a couple of years. Most girls start puberty sometime between 8 and 13 years of age. The first visible signs are breast development and pubic hair. In girls, the growth spurt occurs early in puberty. Growth starts to speed up even as the first signs of puberty appear. In boys, puberty starts a bit later, usually between age 9 and 14. The first visible signs of puberty are pubic hair and growth of the testes (testicles) and penis. Unlike girls, the adolescent growth spurt in boys does not start early in puberty; it occurs a year or two later. In both boys and girls, the growth rate can double during the adolescent growth spurt, increasing from 2 inches per year to 3 or 4 inches per year.

THE END OF GROWTH

The adolescent growth spurt does not last very long. After one to two years of rapid growth, the growth rate starts to slow. By the time a girl has her first menstrual period (typically two years after the start of puberty), the growth rate has usually fallen to approximately 2 inches per year. At this time, the average girl has about 3 inches of growth remaining, but some grow little more than another inch while others grow more than 4. Boys' growth also slows as puberty comes to completion.

Growth does not stop abruptly. The growth rate decreases gradually, dropping from about 3 or 4 inches per year at the peak of the spurt to about 2 inches the next year, then 1 inch per year, then ½ inch. By the time the average girl reaches her 15th birthday and the average boy reaches his 17th, they have less than an inch of growth left. Remember that all these numbers are just approximations, and, as we'll discuss in the next section, the age at which growth tapers off varies widely among individual children. Eventually, however, growth in height does stop completely. In fact, the growth plates disappear from the young man or woman's bones, a process called epiphyseal fusion. Once the growth plates are gone, no further increase in height occurs.

THE RATE OF MATURATION

Different children mature at different rates. Dr. James Tanner, a pioneer in the field of growth research, compared the rate of maturation to a musical tempo. This tempo can affect the child's growth rate, how old he or she looks, when he or she loses baby teeth, and when the child starts puberty.

Some children mature at a slow tempo. These kids often look young for their age and are shorter than average. They go into puberty late and so they have their growth spurt later than most of their peers. When this occurs, the child with the slow pace of maturation feels particularly short because his friends are all shooting up in height. In a year or two, however, the slowly maturing child will begin his growth spurt. By that time, his friends' growth will be slowing down and so the child will start to catch up to his peers. Usually, he will continue to grow after his friends have stopped growing. Some boys with a slow tempo of maturation will still be growing after graduating from high school. Slowly maturing children can end up short, average, or tall as adults.

Other children mature at a rapid tempo. They are often

tall in childhood. They also tend to go into puberty early. The resulting early growth spurt can make them feel very tall compared with their friends. However, these rapidly maturing kids tend to stop growing sooner, at which time their peers tend to catch up. As with slowly maturing kids, the adult height can be tall, average, or even short.

WHAT CONTROLS GROWTH?

Why does one child grow more rapidly than another? Why does one child end up taller than another? Three principal factors regulate a child's growth:

- Genetics
- Nutrition and general health
- Hormones

When a child is not growing at a normal rate, one or more of these three factors are probably responsible. In the next three chapters, we will discuss each of these three factors in some detail.

KEY POINTS TO KEEP IN MIND

Children grow taller because of growth plates present within their bones. Growth is very rapid in early life but decreases with age. This decline is briefly interrupted by the adolescent growth spurt, after which the growth rate again decreases. Growth finally stops in late adolescence, and the growth plates disappear. The tempo of growth and physical maturation varies among different children, with some maturing rapidly and others slowly.

CHAPTER 2

Genetics and Growth

THE INHERITANCE OF STATURE

As most people know from their own experience, height has a strong genetic component. Short parents tend to have short children, and tall parents tend to have tall children. Some people wonder if a boy's height is determined primarily by his father's height whereas a girl's height is determined primarily by her mother's. This turns out not to be true. The height of a child is influenced by the heights of both parents.

You may recall from school that some genetic traits are dominant while others are recessive, and so you might wonder whether tall stature is dominant over short stature or vice versa. In other words, if one parent is tall and the other is short, will the children tend to be short or tall? The answer turns out to be more complicated. Stature is determined by many different genes, and therefore it is neither dominant nor recessive. Each child gets a unique, complex combination of stature-determining genes from his or her parents. If one parent is tall and the other short, the child's stature can be similar to the mother's or the father's, but usually is in between the two. Occasionally, the random assortment of genes can even produce a child who is substantially shorter or taller than both parents.

TARGET HEIGHT

If we know the heights of both parents, we can make an educated guess about the height that their child will attain as an adult. This educated guess is called the target height or adjusted midparental height. Target height can be calculated as follows:

For a boy,

1. *Start with his mother's height.*
2. *Add 5 inches (or 13 cm).*
3. *Then add his father's height.*
4. *Divide by 2.*

For a girl,

1. *Start with her father's height.*
2. *Subtract 5 inches (or 13 cm).*
3. *Then add her mother's height.*
4. *Divide by 2.*

In case you're curious, the 5 inches represents the difference in height between the average man (5 feet, 9½ inches) and the average woman (5 feet, 4½ inches). For a boy, we add 5 inches to his mother's height to take into account the fact that she is female. Adding 5 inches gives us the male equivalent of her height. Then we take that gender-adjusted height and average it with the father's height.

So if a 5-foot, 8-inch man marries a 5-foot, 1-inch woman, we would estimate that their sons would be, on average, about 5 feet, 7 inches (61 inches + 5 inches + 68 inches = 134 inches. 134 ÷ 2 = 67 inches), and we would estimate that their daughters would be, on average, about 5 feet, 2 inches (68 inches − 5 inches + 61 inches = 124 inches. 124 ÷ 2 = 62 inches).

If you are not fond of mathematical formulas, you can use table 2 to convert the parents' height from feet and inches into inches.

Then to determine your child's target height, use table 3 for boys or table 4 for girls.

Look along the left-hand margin of the table to find the father's height. Then look along the top margin of the table to find the mother's height. Follow the column corresponding to the mother's height until it intersects the row corresponding to the father's height. The intersection represents the target height of the child. You can convert back to feet and inches using table 2.

Table 2. Converting Feet-Plus-Inches to Inches

4	feet	4	inches	equals	52	inches
		5	inches		53	
		6	inches		54	
		7	inches		55	
		8	inches		56	
		9	inches		57	
		10	inches		58	
		11	inches		59	
5	feet	0	inches		60	
		1	inches		61	
		2	inches		62	
		3	inches		63	
		4	inches		64	
		5	inches		65	
		6	inches		66	
		7	inches		67	
		8	inches		68	
		9	inches		69	
		10	inches		70	
		11	inches		71	
6	feet	0	inches		72	
		1	inches		73	
		2	inches		74	
		3	inches		75	
		4	inches		76	
		5	inches		77	
		6	inches		78	

Table 3. Calculating Target Height for Boys

Mother's Height in Inches

Father's Height in Inches	54	55	56	57	58	59	60	61	62	63	64	65	66	67	68	69	70
56	57.5	58	58.5	59	59.5	60	60.5	61	61.5	62	62.5	63	63.5	64	64.5	65	65.5
57	58	58.5	59	59.5	60	60.5	61	61.5	62	62.5	63	63.5	64	64.5	65	65.5	66
58	58.5	59	59.5	60	60.5	61	61.5	62	62.5	63	63.5	64	64.5	65	65.5	66	66.5
59	59	59.5	60	60.5	61	61.5	62	62.5	63	63.5	64	64.5	65	65.5	66	66.5	67
60	59.5	60	60.5	61	61.5	62	62.5	63	63.5	64	64.5	65	65.5	66	66.5	67	67.5
61	60	60.5	61	61.5	62	62.5	63	63.5	64	64.5	65	65.5	66	66.5	67	67.5	68
62	60.5	61	61.5	62	62.5	63	63.5	64	64.5	65	65.5	66	66.5	67	67.5	68	68.5
63	61	61.5	62	62.5	63	63.5	64	64.5	65	65.5	66	66.5	67	67.5	68	68.5	69
64	61.5	62	62.5	63	63.5	64	64.5	65	65.5	66	66.5	67	67.5	68	68.5	69	69.5
65	62	62.5	63	63.5	64	64.5	65	65.5	66	66.5	67	67.5	68	68.5	69	69.5	70
66	62.5	63	63.5	64	64.5	65	65.5	66	66.5	67	67.5	68	68.5	69	69.5	70	70.5
67	63	63.5	64	64.5	65	65.5	66	66.5	67	67.5	68	68.5	69	69.5	70	70.5	71
68	63.5	64	64.5	65	65.5	66	66.5	67	67.5	68	68.5	69	69.5	70	70.5	71	71.5
69	64	64.5	65	65.5	66	66.5	67	67.5	68	68.5	69	69.5	70	70.5	71	71.5	72
70	64.5	65	65.5	66	66.5	67	67.5	68	68.5	69	69.5	70	70.5	71	71.5	72	72.5
71	65	65.5	66	66.5	67	67.5	68	68.5	69	69.5	70	70.5	71	71.5	72	72.5	73
72	65.5	66	66.5	67	67.5	68	68.5	69	69.5	70	70.5	71	71.5	72	72.5	73	73.5
73	66	66.5	67	67.5	68	68.5	69	69.5	70	70.5	71	71.5	72	72.5	73	73.5	74
74	66.5	67	67.5	68	68.5	69	69.5	70	70.5	71	71.5	72	72.5	73	73.5	74	74.5
75	67	67.5	68	68.5	69	69.5	70	70.5	71	71.5	72	72.5	73	73.5	74	74.5	75
76	67.5	68	68.5	69	69.5	70	70.5	71	71.5	72	72.5	73	73.5	74	74.5	75	75.5

Table 4. Calculating Target Height for Girls

Father's Height in Inches	Mother's Height in Inches																
	54	55	56	57	58	59	60	61	62	63	64	65	66	67	68	69	70
56	52.5	53	53.5	54	54.5	55	55.5	56	56.5	57	57.5	58	58.5	59	59.5	60	60.5
57	53	53.5	54	54.5	55	55.5	56	56.5	57	57.5	58	58.5	59	59.5	60	60.5	61
58	53.5	54	54.5	55	55.5	56	56.5	57	57.5	58	58.5	59	59.5	60	60.5	61	61.5
59	54	54.5	55	55.5	56	56.5	57	57.5	58	58.5	59	59.5	60	60.5	61	61.5	62
60	54.5	55	55.5	56	56.5	57	57.5	58	58.5	59	59.5	60	60.5	61	61.5	62	62.5
61	55	55.5	56	56.5	57	57.5	58	58.5	59	59.5	60	60.5	61	61.5	62	62.5	63
62	55.5	56	56.5	57	57.5	58	58.5	59	59.5	60	60.5	61	61.5	62	62.5	63	63.5
63	56	56.5	57	57.5	58	58.5	59	59.5	60	60.5	61	61.5	62	62.5	63	63.5	64
64	56.5	57	57.5	58	58.5	59	59.5	60	60.5	61	61.5	62	62.5	63	63.5	64	64.5
65	57	57.5	58	58.5	59	59.5	60	60.5	61	61.5	62	62.5	63	63.5	64	64.5	65
66	57.5	58	58.5	59	59.5	60	60.5	61	61.5	62	62.5	63	63.5	64	64.5	65	65.5
67	58	58.5	59	59.5	60	60.5	61	61.5	62	62.5	63	63.5	64	64.5	65	65.5	66
68	58.5	59	59.5	60	60.5	61	61.5	62	62.5	63	63.5	64	64.5	65	65.5	66	66.5
69	59	59.5	60	60.5	61	61.5	62	62.5	63	63.5	64	64.5	65	65.5	66	66.5	67
70	59.5	60	60.5	61	61.5	62	62.5	63	63.5	64	64.5	65	65.5	66	66.5	67	67.5
71	60	60.5	61	61.5	62	62.5	63	63.5	64	64.5	65	65.5	66	66.5	67	67.5	68
72	60.5	61	61.5	62	62.5	63	63.5	64	64.5	65	65.5	66	66.5	67	67.5	68	68.5
73	61	61.5	62	62.5	63	63.5	64	64.5	65	65.5	66	66.5	67	67.5	68	68.5	69
74	61.5	62	62.5	63	63.5	64	64.5	65	65.5	66	66.5	67	67.5	68	68.5	69	69.5
75	62	62.5	63	63.5	64	64.5	65	65.5	66	66.5	67	67.5	68	68.5	69	69.5	70
76	62.5	63	63.5	64	64.5	65	65.5	66	66.5	67	67.5	68	68.5	69	69.5	70	70.5

Actually, the target height exaggerates the impact of parental height a bit. If the parents are tall, the children tend to be not quite as tall as their target height would predict, and if the parents are short, their children tend to be not quite as short as their target height would predict.

Again, remember that the target height is just a rough estimate. If it were exact, then all the boys in a family would be the same height, as would all the girls, and we know that this is not true. In reality, each child gets a different, random assortment of genes from the parents and so can end up taller or shorter than the parents. The majority of children end up within 2 inches of their target height, but it is not unusual for individual children to end up as much as 4 inches taller or shorter than their target height.

Also, nongenetic factors, such as nutrition, play a role. If a child's nutrition is better than the nutrition her parents received in childhood, then she will probably exceed her target height. On the other hand, if she has a significant illness that interferes with growth, she may not achieve her target height.

ETHNICITY

Certain ethnic groups tend to be tall or short. A striking example is the African Pygmy; adult men are approximately 4 feet, 11 inches, and women approximately 4 feet, 8 inches. For most ethnic groups, the tendency to be tall or short is partly genetic and partly nongenetic. For instance, in the Netherlands the average height for young men is approximately 6 feet, and the average height for young women is approximately 5 feet, 7 inches. This tall stature presumably reflects a favorable environment, including good nutrition and good medical care, and a tall gene pool. In the United States, Caucasian and African Americans have similar heights. Caucasian and African American young men average approximately 5 feet, 10 inches, and young women average approximately 5 feet, 4½ inches. Mexican Americans tend to be shorter. Mexican American young men average approximately 5 feet, 7 inches, and young women approximately 5 feet, 2 inches.

SINGLE GENES THAT CAN AFFECT GROWTH

As we discussed, many genes normally act in combination to determine height. Occasionally, however, a mutation in one single gene can have a powerful influence on growth. Mutations are changes in the DNA sequence. For example, a mutation in one gene (called FGF receptor-3) causes a condition called achondroplasia, in which the growth of the arms and legs is markedly reduced, and the adult height is decreased by about 16 inches. Mutations are often inherited from one or both parents. Specific genetic disorders that cause short stature will be discussed in chapter 7.

CHROMOSOMES AND GROWTH

In addition to mutations in specific growth-determining genes, we know that missing an entire chromosome, as occurs in girls with Turner syndrome, or having an extra chromosome, as occurs in Down syndrome, can have a negative influence on growth. These conditions are discussed in chapter 7.

KEY POINTS TO KEEP IN MIND

Height is influenced by multiple genes. We can use the parents' heights to calculate a child's target height—the height that we would expect the child to attain—but it is just an educated guess. Different ethnic groups tend to be taller or shorter. Occasionally, a mutation in a single gene can strongly affect growth. Although genetics has a powerful effect on growth, it is just half the story. The other half is the environment, that is, the circumstances in which the child is raised.

CHAPTER 3

How Nutrition and Overall Health Affect Growth

Height is not determined entirely by a person's genes. Even a person from a tall family may end up short if he or she does not receive good nutrition or suffers from a serious illness. We cannot change a child's genes, but we can try to optimize his or her nutrition and health. In this chapter, we will explain how nutrition and overall health can affect growth; give you some guidelines as to whether you should be concerned about your child's nutrition; and, if so, suggest some approaches to try to improve nutrition.

HISTORICAL TRENDS IN HEIGHT

You may have noticed that elderly people are, on average, shorter than young adults. Part of this difference arises from the fact that our height actually decreases gradually in later adulthood because our spine can collapse slightly, particularly if we develop osteoporosis. However, not all of the height difference between young and old adults comes from shrinkage. On average, older adults, even when they were young, were never as tall as today's young adults. The average height of adults has gradually increased over the last several hundred years. In the 17th century, the average height of adult men in Europe was probably only about 5 feet, 6 inches, whereas the current average is now close to 5 feet, 10 inches.

Why has height increased over recent centuries? The increase cannot be a result of genetic changes, which require much longer periods of time to occur. Therefore, it must be environmental. (We use the term *environmental* in a general sense to mean anything in our surroundings.) It's hard to be certain about the specific environmental changes responsible, but the change is generally thought to be related to improved nutrition and general health.

Today, most children in the United States do not go to sleep hungry. They eat three meals per day. At each meal, they eat until their hunger is fully satisfied. Furthermore, for most children, the food is not just carbohydrate derived from grain, which is relatively inexpensive, but also contains protein in the form of dairy products and meat. Fruits and vegetables are more abundant than they used to be, even during the winter months. With this abundant and varied food supply, vitamin deficiencies are now less common.

The abundance of food in the United States has largely eliminated severe malnutrition from our society. In fact, we now face an epidemic of obesity. Obesity carries an increased risk for many health problems, but, unlike malnutrition, childhood obesity does not interfere with growth. In fact, obese children tend to be a bit taller than non-obese children, although they end up at a similar adult height.

The trend toward increased height over the past two centuries illustrates the importance of nutrition for growth. In this chapter, we will discuss which types of nutrients are important for growth, why some children do not receive adequate nutrition, and the effects of childhood illness on growth; finally, we explore the practical implications for parents.

WHAT TYPES OF NUTRIENTS ARE IMPORTANT FOR GROWTH?

We do not understand all the nutritional determinants of growth. Much of our current understanding is based only on indirect evidence, such as animal studies or comparing groups of children with different types of diet. However, we think that normal growth requires adequate intake of overall calories, protein, and various micronutrients (vitamins and minerals).

Calories

Overall caloric intake is important. Most of us know about calories because of the opposite problem: Too many calories cause obesity. Calories measure the total energy that our body can extract from food when it is "burned" for energy. We need to burn food to provide the energy for body heat and muscle movement. We even need energy from food just to keep our cells alive and functioning normally. Calories come from three main sources: carbohydrates, proteins, and fats. Fats provide the most calories per gram (9 calories per gram). Carbohydrates and proteins provide fewer (4 calories per gram).

When the body takes in more calories than it burns, the extra chemical energy is stored away for future use, mostly as fat deposits. When the body takes in fewer calories than it burns, it starts to burn up those reserve stores of calories. Children need food energy for all the same reasons that adults need calories and also for one more: They need energy to grow. In children who are not receiving adequate calories, growth slows. In part, it is like a building under construction that has a shortage of bricks. However, the mechanism is actually more complex than that. The body senses the shortage of energy and starts to slow growth as a means of conserving energy. Part of the mechanism probably involves a decrease in the hormone called insulin-like growth factor I (IGF-I), which comes in part from the liver and is very important for growth. IGF-I production is controlled both by growth hormone from the pituitary gland, and also by nutrition. When a child is undernourished, IGF-I levels drop and growth slows. Presumably, the body does this to conserve nutrients for vital functions. In times of famine, growth is a luxury that must be postponed until better days.

Protein

Protein is important for growth in two ways. First, as mentioned in the previous section, proteins, along with carbohydrates and fats, can provide calories. In other words, proteins can be burned as a source of energy. Second, proteins also provide important raw materials to build new tissues.

Proteins consist of chains of smaller molecules called amino acids. When you eat foods containing plant or animal proteins, these proteins are broken down into amino acids in the intestines, absorbed into the bloodstream, and distributed to every cell in the body, where they can be reassembled into human proteins. These human proteins are required for many different kinds of functions in cells. They are used, for example, as enzymes to guide chemical reactions, as hormones to signal from one cell to another, as antibodies to fight infection, as a structural scaffolding for bones, and as a mechanical motor to contract muscles.

If children receive adequate overall calories but markedly inadequate protein, they develop a condition known as kwashiorkor. You may have seen pictures of children from developing countries with kwashiorkor. They often have distended abdomens and many health problems in addition to growth failure. Kwashiorkor is fortunately now rare in the United States. However, less severe protein deficiency may also impair growth.

Most US children do take in adequate protein, which can be derived from animal sources including meat, fish, dairy products, and egg whites; it can also come from plant sources, such as grains, seeds, nuts, and beans. However, some plant sources may not provide all the kinds of amino acids needed by the body. If your child is a vegetarian or, for other reasons, is not receiving a normal amount of dairy products and meat, we suggest that you talk to his or her physician to determine whether your child is receiving an adequate quantity and quality of protein. The physician may refer you to a dietitian who may have you record your child's intake and can then calculate whether protein is adequate in both quality and quantity.

Unlike protein, the quality and quantity of carbohydrate and fat in the diet are not as critical for growth, as long as the total intake of calories is adequate. There is some evidence that your choice of fats (for example, saturated versus unsaturated) and your choice of carbohydrates (simple sugars versus complex carbohydrates) may have other health implications, but they do not have recognized effects on growth.

Micronutrients (Vitamins and Minerals)

Carbohydrates, proteins, and fats are referred to as macronutrients because they are needed in relatively large quantities. Vitamins and minerals are referred to as micronutrients because they are needed only in relatively small amounts. For most vitamins, you need less than one thousandth of an ounce per day to stay healthy.

Vitamins are organic molecules that our bodies cannot produce by themselves (except for vitamin D, which we can manufacture if we get enough sunlight). We need to take vitamins into our body by eating food from a plant or animal that can produce the vitamin molecule. Vitamins can also be produced commercially and added either to a vitamin pill or to food. Milk today is supplemented with vitamins A and D, for instance, and many breakfast cereals are fortified with multiple vitamins.

Minerals are inorganic molecules such as iron, calcium, and zinc. Like vitamins, we can obtain minerals from certain foods. As you probably know, meat is a source of iron, and milk is a source of calcium. Many vitamin pills contain certain minerals in addition to vitamins. Also, it is possible to obtain specific minerals from fortified foods like some breakfast cereals.

It is important that children receive adequate vitamins and minerals for their overall health as well as for growth. In certain developing countries, for example, there is evidence that zinc deficiency can impair growth. In the United States, vitamin and mineral deficiencies are less common but still exist. Iron deficiency is not uncommon, particularly in infants; vitamin D deficiency is still found, particularly in infants with dark skin who are being breast-fed, and in northern climates where there is less sunlight. These deficiencies may have important health consequences.

For most American children receiving a normal, reasonable, well-balanced diet, however, vitamin and mineral deficiencies are not thought to be a common cause of short stature. Consequently, most physicians will not suggest vitamin supplements for children with short stature unless there is some specific reason, such as a restricted diet or an intestinal problem causing the child not to absorb vitamins normally.

FOOD BELIEFS

Sometimes, nutrition can be inadequate because the family has certain beliefs or preferences related to food. For example, if a family is vegan and avoids all meat, fish, eggs, and dairy products, the children may not be receiving enough high-quality protein unless a special effort is made to address this problem. Vegan families may also need to be careful about receiving certain micronutrients such as vitamin B_{12} and iron. Another example is a family trying to avoid excess weight gain by minimizing calories, fat, and/or carbohydrates. Perhaps dinner consists only of a salad. These sorts of diets may be appropriate for adults trying to lose weight, but they can interfere with growth in a child. Sometimes children may hear their parents discussing diets and take on inappropriate concerns about their own diet. A fear of obesity can limit children's food intake and cause growth problems. Other children may develop certain harmful ideas about food from sources other than the parents. Some children who are not overweight may be trying to limit their food intake to perform well in athletics or dance. One patient of ours was a boy who wanted to stay in a particular weight class in wrestling. He was limiting his food intake to avoid gaining weight. Once he understood that his food avoidance was actually stunting his growth, he began to eat more and his growth improved.

EATING DISORDERS

When a child's eating behavior represents a potential threat to health, we say that he or she has an eating disorder. Eating disorders include anorexia nervosa and bulimia. In the former, the child or adult typically refuses to take in enough food to maintain a normal body weight. Individuals with anorexia nervosa are usually intensely afraid of gaining weight. They often have a disturbed body perception; they think they are overweight even though they are underweight. One 12-year-old girl, for example, was a little overweight and was occasionally teased. She began to lose weight—and didn't stop. She became quite thin and still thought she was too fat. She loved to prepare food for other people, but she ate little herself. Her parents became worried and brought her to the pediatrician. The girl had anorexia nervosa and needed both psychological and behavioral therapy.

Bulimic patients typically have episodes of binge eating and inappropriate compensatory methods to prevent weight gain. Binge eating means a sudden increase in food intake; individuals often eat a large amount in an hour or two. To try to compensate for the binge, the person may induce vomiting or take a laxative or diuretic.

Often, children with eating disorders will attempt to hide the problem. If you are concerned that your child might have anorexia nervosa, bulimia, or another eating disorder, talk to your child's doctor.

PICKY EATERS

Some children are just picky eaters. They may have a very limited number of foods that they will eat. Some kids want to live on peanut butter and jelly sandwiches or macaroni and cheese. If your child is like this, talk to your pediatrician about strategies to improve the variety of foods they'll eat. Sometimes your doctor may also suggest a multivitamin pill or other nutritional supplements.

Some children have a disorder in chewing or swallowing food or an oral aversion to foods of certain textures. These children may need to be referred to a program that specializes in childhood feeding disorders. Occasionally, children may avoid certain foods because they cannot digest them well due to a gastrointestinal problem.

Other kids just don't want to eat much. You place a big plate of food in front of your child for dinner, but he takes three bites and says he is full. On the other hand, some parents have unrealistic expectations of how much their child should eat. If a child is a normal height and weight and growing well, then he or she is probably taking in enough calories. But if a child is gaining weight and/or height poorly, the calories might be inadequate. If your child is a picky eater and short and/or noticeably thin, discuss your concerns about nutrition with his or her doctor.

MEDICATIONS AND APPETITE

Appetite can be suppressed by some medications. For example, many of the medications used to treat attention deficit disorder (also known as ADD, ADHD, or "hyperactivity") can impair appetite. If your child is on any medication, especially one for attention deficit disorder, and has problems with height or weight, you should discuss the problem with your child's physician. If the physician agrees that the medication may be to blame, he or she may be able to adjust the dose or change to a different medication. Sometimes, however, some suppression of appetite may have to be tolerated in order to allow the child to learn well in school. In such difficult cases, you may want to consult a specialist, such as a child psychiatrist or other physician with particular expertise in this condition.

CHRONIC ILLNESS

Children often grow poorly because of a chronic (long-lasting) illness. Such a chronic illness may involve essentially any part of the body, including the heart, lungs, intestinal tract, liver, kidneys—and might spring from almost any cause, including genetic mutations, infectious agents, autoimmunity, cancer, or birth defects. Much of the effect of chronic illnesses on growth may be caused by nutritional problems. Many illnesses cause children to suffer from a poor appetite. In addition, children with diseases of the gastrointestinal tract may not absorb nutrients prop-

erly. However, some illnesses also impair growth for reasons other than nutrition. In kidney failure, for example,
metabolic wastes—normally cleared by the kidneys—
build up and interfere with growing cells. Also,
inflammation (the body's response to tissue injury), which
occurs with many types of illnesses, may interfere with
growth.

If your child has a chronic illness that is interfering
with growth, the most important thing to do is make sure
that he or she is receiving good medical care for the underlying illness. If you are concerned that the care is not
optimal, you may wish to seek a second opinion. It is often helpful to seek the opinion of a specialist. For example, if your child has severe asthma, you may wish to have
him or her evaluated by a pediatric pulmonologist (lung
specialist).

The physician caring for your child should be keeping
an eye on the weight and height curves (which we'll discuss
in later chapters); these can sometimes be a useful indicator of the severity of the illness and the effectiveness of
treatment. If you are concerned about your child's growth,
discuss it with your child's pediatrician and any other physician caring for the chronic illness.

When a child with a chronic illness is not receiving
adequate nutrition, the medical team and the parents will
often work hard to try to improve intake through dietary
counseling, nutritional supplements, changing medications, or even inserting a tube into the stomach or giving
the nutrition intravenously. In such cases, nutrition can

be critical for the child's ability to withstand the illness. In very ill children, the issue of growth may be far less important than other health concerns, but the growth pattern may still serve as a useful clue to physicians about the child's nutritional status.

SUBTLE DISEASE AND SUBTLE NUTRITIONAL DEFICIENCY

As we will discuss in chapters 7 and 8, when a child is growing unusually slowly but does not have any obvious other signs of disease, a physician should still look carefully for some hidden illness or nutritional problem that might be interfering with growth. Often, however, no underlying illness is found. The child may be short because of genetics or for unknown reasons. In this situation, we may wonder whether subtle nutritional problems may still be playing a role in the decreased growth. It is true that many of the children who are growing poorly for unclear reasons tend to be thin, and parents report that they are picky eaters. It's hard to know whether these children are growing slowly because they're not eating well, or if they aren't eating well because they are growing slowly, so that their bodies need fewer calories.

SO WHAT'S A PARENT TO DO?

Parents often want to know whether they should change a short child's diet, encourage the child to eat more, and/or give a vitamin pill. The answer depends on the cause of the short stature and the child's individual circumstances.

If the short stature is primarily a nutritional issue, then a change in nutrition is obviously important. Remember the boy mentioned earlier who was avoiding weight gain because of wrestling. In his case, it took only a simple explanation that his poor food intake was stunting his growth. He started gaining weight and growing better. For the girl we mentioned with anorexia nervosa, it was not so easy to correct the problem. She was seen in a clinic specializing in eating disorders. She has gained weight, but the anorexia remains a serious ongoing problem.

What about the typical child with short stature that is not due to any recognized medical problem? Perhaps one or both of the parents are also short. There are some clues that nutrition might be playing a role for certain of these children. For example, many children with short stature do appear thin and have a mildly low IGF-I level in their blood, which might be caused by mild undernutrition. On the other hand, there isn't really much rigorous scientific evidence that nutritional intervention will help their growth.

So what should you do? We suggest that you try your best to provide good nutrition for your child. After all, even when growth isn't an issue, good nutrition is still a worthwhile goal for general health. Try to ensure that your child receives a variety of healthy foods including adequate calories, protein, vitamins, and minerals. In particular, strive to have your child eat reasonable servings of protein (especially meat, fish, poultry, egg whites, or dairy products) each day. One useful guide to good nutrition is the US Department of Agriculture (USDA) Food Guide Pyramid (www.mypyramid.gov). It suggests reasonable daily amounts of carbohydrates, vegetables, fruits, dairy products, and meats.

For children who are picky eaters and don't get a good variety of foods, try to gradually increase their list of acceptable foods. Even if they decline most new foods at first, keep offering a variety of healthy, nutritious foods at meals. Younger children especially may be modeling their behavior after yours, so they should see you eating and enjoying the same variety of healthy foods.

For children who are short but don't appear thin, we don't suggest pushing an increased overall food intake, particularly for children who are short but overweight for their height. In this case, just try to be sure that they get a good variety of foods. However, if your child is unusually short and is thin, you probably wish you could increase overall food intake—that is, total calories. Certainly, you can try to avoid skipped or rushed meals. You can offer foods that contain plenty of calories (carbohydrate, fat, and protein). Still, in the same way that overweight people find it hard to eat less than their appetite dictates, underweight people often find it hard to eat more than their appetite dictates. Many nutrition experts believe that it's a mistake to punish, reward, or coerce your child to eat more, and that these interactions can sometimes worsen problems. If you find yourself battling your child over food, something has gone wrong, and you should talk to your pediatrician about other approaches.

Some parents wonder whether junk food will stunt their child's growth. Well, foods such as soda, candy, and potato chips are considered "empty calories" in that they provide calories but little by way of vitamins, minerals, fiber, protein, or other valuable nutrients. These sorts of foods should be limited in most children, especially those who are overweight. However, they are not specifically a problem for growth. As long as a short child is receiving a good variety of foods in general, junk foods will not specifically interfere with growth. In fact, for the short, skinny child, you probably need not be quite as strict about these foods as you would for an overweight child.

If your child is short and you are concerned that his or her diet might not be adequate, discuss this issue with your child's physician, particularly if your child has a chronic illness, if your family has specific dietary practices (say, vegetarian or vegan), or if your child just will not eat a good variety or quantity of food. If your physician thinks there is reason for concern, you may be referred to a dietitian, who will probably have you keep a food diary. The dietitian will then calculate your child's intake of calories and specific nutrients. If your physician believes that your child's nutritional intake is inadequate in some way, he or she may counsel you to change your child's diet or perhaps add a multivitamin or other nutritional supplement. Understand, however, that most children need nothing more than a reasonable variety of healthy foods.

We also caution you against food faddism and poorly substantiated claims from companies that sell nutritional supplements. Many of the unusual diets and nutritional supplements on the market have not, despite claims in their advertising, been adequately tested for safety and efficacy. You may have seen advertisements for supplements that claim to be "growth hormone releasers." These supplements may contain certain amino acids such as arginine; when taken in large amounts by an intravenous infusion, these substances *will* cause the pituitary gland to release a brief burst of growth hormone. However, there is no evidence that such supplements, taken chronically by mouth, have any sustained effect on growth. We recommend that you talk to your child's physician about any nutritional intervention you may be considering.

Even if you can get a child with short stature to eat better, don't expect a miraculous growth spurt. As we mentioned earlier, in the United States relatively few cases of short stature are due to nutritional deficiency. But good nutrition is a worthwhile lifelong goal and may help optimize growth for some children. For additional information on childhood nutrition, see the *American Academy of Pediatrics Guide to Your Child's Nutrition,* mentioned in "Selected References" at the end of this book.

KEY POINTS TO KEEP IN MIND

To grow optimally, children require good nutrition, including adequate intake of overall calories, protein, and micronutrients (vitamins and minerals). Growth is also affected by the overall health of the child. These effects probably explain the overall increase in human height seen over the past several centuries and the decreased growth seen in impoverished regions of the world. In the United States today, some children have inadequate nutrition because of certain food beliefs or practices, actual eating disorders, chronic illnesses, or medications. Other children are just picky eaters or seem to have a poor appetite. If your child is short and you are concerned that he or she is not receiving adequate nutrition, you should consult his or her physician. For children who have not been receiving adequate quality or quantity of food, improvements in nutrition can improve growth.

CHAPTER 4

Hormones and Growth

So far we've discussed the important effects of genetics, nutrition, and general health on childhood growth, but there's one more important set of factors to consider—hormones. Even a child from a tall family who is well nourished and in good general health may be extremely short if he or she has a hormonal abnormality. You probably know that growth hormone is important for normal growth—and it is—but, in addition, insulin-like growth factor I, thyroid hormone, cortisol, androgens, and estrogens also have important effects on growth. In this chapter, we will discuss the powerful effects of these hormones and how abnormalities can cause growth disorders.

HORMONES

Hormones are chemical messengers that help coordinate activities of different organs in the body and coordinate the response of the body to its surroundings. Most hormones are produced in one of the endocrine glands such as the pituitary gland, thyroid gland, adrenal gland, testes (testicles), or ovaries (see figure 2). Each of these endocrine glands produces different hormones. The hormone enters the bloodstream, where it is distributed throughout the body. Hormones then act on various other organs to perform their functions.

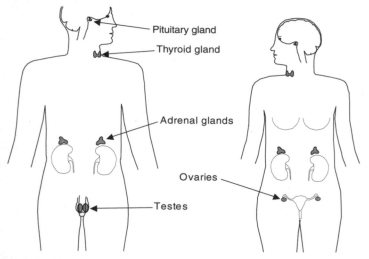

Figure 2. Diagram showing the locations of certain endocrine (hormone-producing) glands. The female has all the same endocrine glands except that she has ovaries instead of testes.

Six hormones are most important for growth: growth hormone, insulin-like growth factor I , thyroid hormone, cortisol, androgen, and estrogen. Abnormal levels—either increased or decreased—of these hormones can cause significant growth problems (see table 5).

Table 5. Major Hormones That Regulate Growth

Hormone	Source	Effect on Growth
Growth hormone	Pituitary gland	Accelerates growth
Insulin-like growth factor I	Liver primarily	Accelerates growth
Thyroid hormone	Thyroid gland	Accelerates growth
Cortisol	Adrenal gland	Slows growth in height but causes weight gain
Androgen	Testes, adrenal gland, ovaries	Accelerates growth
Estrogen	Ovaries, testes	Accelerates growth but also causes it to stop earlier

GROWTH HORMONE: OF MUNCHKINS AND GIANTS

As its name suggests, growth hormone (GH) is a powerful regulator of childhood growth. Growth hormone is produced in the pituitary gland, a pea-size organ located underneath the brain (see figure 2). Signals from a nearby part of the brain called the hypothalamus control the pituitary gland. The pituitary gland produces not just growth hormone but multiple hormones that affect health in many ways. The pituitary is sometimes referred to as the master endocrine gland because it makes hormones that control other endocrine glands, including the thyroid gland, the adrenal gland, the testes, and the ovaries.

Growth hormone is produced by the pituitary gland in pulses, most of which occur at night. The hormone enters the bloodstream and is carried throughout the body. Some travels to the liver, where it causes the liver cells to make a second hormone, insulin-like growth factor I (abbreviated IGF-I). GH and IGF-I act throughout the body to stimulate growth. For example, they act on the cartilage cells of the growth plates in the bones, speeding their growth, causing the bones to grow longer, and consequently causing the child's height to increase.

Growth Hormone Deficiency

If a child's body cannot make growth hormone, growth will be severely impaired. Children with complete growth hormone deficiency are usually normal in size at birth but grow slowly during infancy and childhood, resulting in severe short stature. However, complete growth hormone deficiency is rare; partial deficiency is more common. Partial deficiency causes a milder impairment in growth.

Unlike some other causes of growth failure, people with growth hormone deficiency have fairly normal body proportions; growth of the arms, legs, and trunk is affected similarly. These individuals tend to be chubby and have high-pitched voices. Many of the actors who played Munchkins in the movie *The Wizard of Oz* probably had growth hormone deficiency. It is uncommon to see individuals looking like this in the United States today because most children with severe growth hormone deficiency are treated with growth hormone. Most of the extraordinarily short adults that you see in the media and in everyday life today have altered body proportions—typically, short limbs with a relatively large head and trunk. These individuals do not have growth hormone deficiency but rather a skeletal dys-plasia, which is a genetic problem affecting the growth plates within the bones (discussed in chapters 2 and 7).

Growth hormone has other functions, aside from stim-ulating growth. For example, it tends to reduce body fat and increase muscle tissue. As a result, even adults who develop growth hormone deficiency can have problems, including increased body fat and decreased muscle mass.

Growth hormone deficiency will be discussed in more detail in chapter 10.

Growth Hormone Excess

Occasionally, a child will produce too much growth hormone, usually because of a tumor in the pituitary gland. As you might guess, excess growth hormone can cause extraordinary growth. This condition, called pitu-itary gigantism, is very rare. The most famous case of pi-tuitary gigantism is a man named Robert Pershing Wadlow, who became known as the Alton Giant because he grew up in Alton, Illinois. Mr. Wadlow was born in 1918 at a normal weight, but by 18 months of age he weighed 62 pounds. By the age of eight, he was 6 feet, 2 inches, tall and weighed 195 pounds. He eventually attained a height of 8 feet, 11 inches. Unfortunately, Mr. Wadlow experi-enced serious health problems caused by growth hormone excess. These side effects serve as a reminder that we should not use growth hormone treatment indiscrimi-nately or excessively. These side effects will be discussed in chapter 11.

Growth Hormone in Adults

Although adult bodies continue to manufacture growth hormone, the hormone can only increase height during childhood and adolescence. Once the growth plates in the bones disappear, normally in late adolescence (see chapter 1), growth hormone can no longer increase height. However, adults who develop growth hormone excess (a condition called acromegaly) or deficiency do experience medical problems because the hormone also affects the body in ways unrelated to growth.

THYROID HORMONE

Thyroid hormone is produced by the thyroid gland, located in the front of the neck (see figure 2). This hormone has major effects on many organs and functions in the body. You can think of it as a message that says, *Speed up*. Thyroid hormone speeds the heart rate. It speeds the rate of metabolism, causing you to burn calories faster. It speeds movement of the bowels. It even causes the brain to "speed up."

Occasionally, the thyroid gland can make too much thyroid hormone. When this occurs, people often have an increased heart rate. They may lose weight despite an increased appetite because they are burning up calories rapidly. They often feel warm even when the temperature in the room is comfortable for others. They can have diarrhea. They often feel nervous and shaky. This condition, known as hyperthyroidism, can have serious health consequences.

It can occur in children, but will not be discussed further because it is not a major cause of growth problems. On the other hand, deficiency of thyroid hormone is an important cause of short stature.

Hypothyroidism

Sometimes, the thyroid gland does not produce enough thyroid hormone, leading to decreased thyroid hormone levels in the blood. As you might imagine, this condition, known as hypothyroidism, causes the body to slow down in many ways. Often the heart rate is decreased, although this may be mild. Some hypothyroid individuals feel cold much of the time, even when others in the same room are comfortable. Their appetite is typically decreased, yet they may gain weight because they are burning calories more slowly. They may have constipation. Those with hypothyroidism may think and act more slowly than is normal for them, although children with hypothyroidism often do well in school. Hypothyroid individuals often complain of fatigue and a lack of energy. Their hair may be coarse, and their skin dry. Not all hypothyroid individuals will feel all these symptoms. Conversely, many people with some of these symptoms do not have hypothyroidism.

Hypothyroidism is usually caused by some problem within the thyroid gland itself. At other times, however, the thyroid gland is itself normal, but it is not receiving the right signal from the pituitary gland. Normally, the pituitary produces a hormone called thyroid stimulating hormone (TSH), which stimulates the thyroid gland to make thyroid hormone. If the pituitary gland fails to make enough TSH, hypothyroidism results.

Hypothyroidism can be congenital or acquired. In congenital hypothyroidism, the thyroid hormone deficiency is present at birth. Usually congenital hypothyroidism is picked up by newborn screening programs. You may recall that blood was obtained from your child's heel in his or her first few days of life. The blood was absorbed onto a paper card and then sent to the state lab, where it was screened for many congenital diseases, including hypothyroidism. These programs identify most kids with congenital hypothyroidism, which is important because untreated congenital hypothyroidism can cause mental retardation. However, the screening programs will on rare occasions miss a child with congenital hypothyroidism. Also, if your child was born in another country, he or she may not have received this test.

In children with congenital hypothyroidism, birth size is usually normal, but growth is often impaired beginning in infancy. Infants with congenital hypothyroidism may also have a hoarse cry, a large fontanel (soft spot on the top of the head), large tongue, dry skin, poor muscle tone, jaundice (yellow skin color from too much bilirubin) that lasts more than a week, constipation, decreased activity, difficulty feeding, cool skin, and an umbilical hernia. As with hypothyroidism in later life, not all patients have obvious physical signs of the disease, which is one of the reasons that newborn screening is so important.

Other children develop hypothyroidism at some point after birth. This condition, termed acquired hypothyroidism, will be discussed in chapter 7.

CORTISOL

Cortisol is a hormone produced by the adrenal glands, which lie just above the kidneys (see figure 2). Cortisol is sometimes known as a stress hormone because physical and psychological stress causes an increase in its secretion.

Cortisol has complex effects on many different parts of the body. Cortisol deficiency can cause poor appetite or even nausea and vomiting, weight loss, and fatigue. While it can be fatal if not treated, it's not a common cause of short stature. On the other hand, cortisol excess is one of the recognized causes of short stature.

Cushing Syndrome

Excess cortisol causes a disorder known as Cushing syndrome (named for Harvey Cushing, an eminent neurosurgeon who contributed to our understanding of this condition). In adults, it can include a wide variety of signs and symptoms, including weight gain, purple stretch marks, weakness, easy bruising, high blood pressure, osteoporosis, and/or sleep disturbance. In children, many of the same manifestations occur, but in addition they will have slowing of growth in height despite excessive weight gain. Therefore, on the growth chart, they may cross over to lower height percentiles and higher weight percentiles.

If a child has had Cushing syndrome for a while, he or she might even be below the 5th percentile for height but above the 95th percentile for weight.

Cushing syndrome is not always caused by excess cortisol secretion from the adrenal glands. Sometimes it is caused by medications. Medications that cause Cushing syndrome are properly referred to as glucocorticoids, though they are often just called steroids. This term is less precise because *steroids* is a general term that includes many chemicals, not just cortisol and other glucocorticoids, but also androgens (including those androgens abused by athletes), estrogens, and other natural and medicinal chemicals with a similar chemical structure. Glucocorticoids are steroids that act in the body like cortisol. Many doctors also refer to these medications by a third name, corticosteroids, and we will use that term in the remainder of the book. Cushing syndrome caused by taking large doses of corticosteroids will be discussed in chapter 7.

ESTROGEN

Estrogen is sometimes referred to as the female hormone. In women, it is produced primarily by the ovaries (see figure 2). The principal estrogen made by the body is called estradiol. Estrogen levels are low in young girls—for example, at five years of age. These levels increase during puberty, however, causing growth of the breasts and subsequently menstruation. Estrogens are also present in adolescent boys and adult men, although in lower concentrations than in females. In males, the estrogen is produced in the body primarily by the chemical conversion of androgens into estrogens. Some medications, such as birth control pills, also contain estrogens.

Estrogens have a dual effect on growth. First, they accelerate growth. This effect is partly indirect: Estrogens increase growth hormone secretion from the pituitary gland, which then secondarily accelerates growth. The adolescent growth spurt in girls is primarily due to estrogens, secreted by the ovaries beginning at puberty. Even in boys, much of the adolescent growth spurt is due to estrogens. At puberty, the testes begin to increase production of testosterone. Some of the testosterone is converted into estradiol, which accelerates growth. However, some of the growth spurt in boys may also be due to the direct effects of the testosterone that is not converted to estrogen.

The second effect of estrogen is to hasten the end of growth by acting on the growth plates, the structures in the bones that are responsible for growth in height. As discussed in chapter 1, in infancy the growth plates are very active, causing rapid growth. Gradually, though, they become less active, causing growth to slow. Eventually, in late adolescence, they stop functioning altogether and disappear from the bones in the process called epiphyseal fusion. Although estrogen temporarily speeds the rate of growth, it also speeds the aging process in the growth plates. As a result, estrogen causes the growth plates to run out of steam sooner. Consequently, growth will stop sooner, and epiphyseal fusion will occur sooner. This effect of estrogen, to hasten the end of growth, is not sudden. It occurs over months and years.

Thus, estrogen has two effects on growth, one positive and one negative. It speeds growth but also hastens the end of growth. You might wonder what the net effect is on the eventual adult height—is the positive effect more important than the negative, leading to a net increase? In fact, it turns out that the negative effect predominates. Estrogens speed up growth in the short term, but because growth stops sooner the final adult height will be decreased.

We know that the net effect of estrogen is negative from several different observations. First, there are rare children who develop puberty at a very early age. High estrogen levels cause these children to grow rapidly at first, so that they are temporarily taller than their peers. After some years, however, these children stop growing before their peers, and they will be, on average, short as adults. Fortunately, we now have medication to stop this process. Second, there are rare children who do not go into puberty at all on their own and need to be given medication to induce it. If puberty is not induced at the normal age, these children are often shorter than normal during their teenage years because all of their peers are experiencing growth spurts. Still, once the problem in these children is understood and puberty is finally induced with medications, they end up, on average, tall as adults. This effect is even more striking in a few rare individuals who cannot make estrogen or cannot respond to estrogen because of a genetic abnormality. These patients continue to grow slowly into young adulthood and eventually can end up very tall.

Because estrogen has a net negative effect on adult height, endocrinologists have considered blocking its production in order to increase adult height. One way to do this is to shut off puberty. Medications have been developed to do this. This approach will be discussed in chapter 11.

ANDROGENS

Androgens are sometimes referred to as male hormones. In men, they are produced primarily by the testes (also known as testicles). In boys under 10 years old— androgen levels are low. These levels increase during puberty, causing growth of body hair, enlargement of the penis, deepening of the voice, acne, increased muscle mass, and behavioral changes. Androgens are also present in adolescent girls and women, but at lower levels than in males.

Many specific chemicals, both natural and synthetic, can act as androgens. The most important androgen made by the human body is testosterone. In addition, many synthetic androgens are used as medications. Androgens are also abused by some athletes. In this context, they are often referred to as anabolic steroids.

Androgens stimulate growth in two ways. The body can convert many of them into estrogens, which stimulate growth; androgens can also stimulate bone growth directly.

KEY POINTS TO KEEP IN MIND

Growth is regulated by multiple hormones. Growth hormone, which is made in the pituitary gland, stimulates growth, partly by increasing liver production of another hormone, IGF-I. Consequently, growth hormone deficiency can cause marked short stature. Thyroid hormone is also important for normal growth, and thus hypothyroidism is another important cause of growth failure. Cortisol, which comes from the adrenal glands, inhibits growth. Therefore, overproduction of cortisol by the adrenal gland or taking large doses of cortisol-like medications causes growth failure. Estrogen stimulates growth in the short term but also hastens the end of growth in the long term. The net effect of estrogen on adult height is negative. Androgens also stimulate growth.

CHAPTER 5

Is My Child's Growth Normal?

In chapters 1 through 4, we tried to explain some of the key concepts about how children grow. With these concepts in mind, we can get down to more practical matters. One of the first questions parents ask is, *Is my child's growth normal?* The answer is not as simple as it might seem. To address it we need to know the child's height accurately. We then plot the child's height and weight on a growth chart. The growth chart tells us the child's height and weight percentiles. If we have multiple points plotted over time, we can assess the overall pattern of growth. Then, to decide if a child's growth is normal, we consider the child's height and weight percentiles, the overall pattern of growth, the family background, and the child's health. It sounds complicated, but it should become clearer as we explain each step.

HEIGHT MEASUREMENT IN
THE DOCTOR'S OFFICE

To know if your child's height is normal or not, we first need to know your child's height accurately. Unfortunately, accurate height measurement is not as easy or as common as you might think.

Different doctors use different techniques to measure height, some more accurate than others. The most precise technique involves standing the child with the heels, buttocks, shoulders, and back of the head touching a wall. The person making the measurement asks the child to stand up very straight. A horizontal bar is then lowered to touch the top of the child's head. A device used to measure height in this way is called a stadiometer.

Unfortunately many health care providers do not use stadiometers to measure height. Instead, some use a device attached to a scale so that weight and height can be measured with the same piece of equipment. Measurements using these devices usually do not involve a wall or other vertical surface to keep the child straight. Often the swinging bar placed on the child's head is not horizontal.

For children younger than two or three, standing heights are not accurate even with the best equipment. In this case, we measure the child's length while he or she is lying down, faceup. This measurement is called supine length. The most accurate way to measure supine length is to use a device on which a child can be placed horizontally with the head touching a perpendicular surface. The child's legs are then extended fully and a sliding plate is brought flat against the bottom of the child's foot. Some physicians' offices do not have this equipment; instead, the child's length may be measured by placing him or her on a piece of paper, making a mark at the head and foot, and then measuring the distance between the two marks. This technique is less accurate.

Sometimes specific errors are made in length or height measurements, particularly if the person doing the measurement is inexperienced. For example, some children have their height measured with shoes on. If the measurement gives a surprising or worrisome result, ask for it to be repeated. If the two measurements agree, the result is more likely to be accurate. If they disagree, one or more additional measurements should be done.

In clinics that specialize in growth problems (pediatric endocrinology clinics), height measurements are usually made with a stadiometer by an experienced nurse or by the endocrinologist. Often two or more measurements will be made initially; if these do not agree closely, additional measurements are performed.

Most children have their height and weight measured in their doctor's office whenever they come in for a routine health checkup, which means that growth measurements are usually done frequently in the first couple of years of life and thereafter generally once per year. In children who are growing slowly, the doctor may make measurements more frequently.

HEIGHT MEASUREMENTS AT HOME

All children should be seen by a physician or other health care provider for regular health care visits that include measurements of height and weight. In addition, many families like to make measurements at home, often marking the child's height on a wall once or twice a year. With the proper techniques, these home measurements can actually be quite accurate. Because older children usually go to see their physicians less often than younger, home measurements can supplement the occasional ones done at the doctor's office and often can provide reassurance that the child is growing normally. Instructions for making these measurements can be found in appendix A.

For children less than two years old, standing heights are not accurate, and so we measure body length with the child lying down. Unfortunately, this measurement of supine length is a bit trickier than measuring standing height. Instructions for measuring supine length are found in appendix B. For children between their second and third birthdays, you can measure either the standing height or the supine length.

If you are making home measurements, we suggest you do it with a positive attitude. You and your child can enjoy seeing the height marks steadily climb up the wall. You do not want to send a message to your child that height is crucial in life or that there is something wrong with him or her. We'll talk more about these important psychological issues in chapter 8.

GROWTH CHARTS

To determine whether your child's height and weight are normal, your child's health care provider will usually plot the height and weight on a growth chart—a graph of height and weight versus age. The growth chart will show where your child's height and weight fall relative to normal children of the same age. When you take your child to the health care provider for routine visits, you can ask to see the growth chart and discuss your child's growth pattern.

In addition, if you are handy with graphs, you can plot the height and weight measurements you do at home on a growth chart yourself. Growth charts are printed in appendix C along with detailed instructions for plotting height and weight. If you have any previous measurements, plot them on the same growth chart.

Interpreting a growth chart well requires experience, so you should not make any medical decisions based on your own interpretation. Instead, discuss the growth chart with your child's health care provider. If you understand some of the principles of interpretation, you will interact with your child's health care provider more knowledgeably.

Height and Weight Percentiles

Notice the curves on the growth chart that represent the different percentiles for height and weight. Determine whether your child's points fall on one of the curves or between two curves, or below the 3rd percentile, or above the 97th percentile. A sample growth chart is shown in figure 3 on the facing page. This is the height growth chart for boys, age 2 through 20. As an example, imagine that a 10½-year-old boy has a height of 54¼ inches. His height would plot out at the x mark, and we would say that his height is between the 25th and 50th percentiles. As another example, imagine that a 5¾-year-old boy is 41 inches tall. His height would plot out at the + mark, and we would say that his height is just below the 3rd percentile. By the way, the growth charts provided here may look different from those your pediatrician uses. There are many different versions. For example, some growth charts do not have a 3rd percentile curve; their lowest depicted curve is the 5th percentile.

The percentile tells you where your child's height or weight falls compared with other children his or her age. A girl at the 5th percentile for height is taller than 5 percent of girls her age and shorter than 95 percent of girls her age. A boy at the 3rd percentile is taller than 3 percent of boys his age and shorter than 97 percent. A boy at the 50th percentile is average in that he is taller than 50 percent of boys his age and shorter than 50 percent.

WHAT PERCENTILES ARE NORMAL?

Generally when we say *normal,* we mean approximately between the 3rd and the 97th percentiles, but remember that this is a statistical definition. Just because children fall outside this range doesn't necessarily mean that their height or weight is a problem. It just means that their height is

CDC Growth Charts: United States

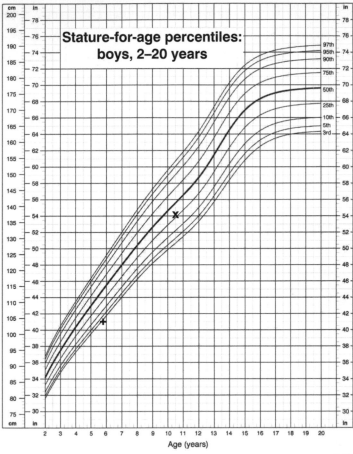

Figure 3. Height growth chart for boys age 2–20 years. The x mark represents a 10½-year-old boy with a height of 54¼ inches. His height is between the 25th and 50th percentiles. The + mark represents a 5¾-year-old boy who is 41 inches tall. His height is just below the 3rd percentile.

different from most children their age. Conversely, if your child's height and weight fall within the normal range, it does not guarantee that there is no growth problem. For example, sometimes a child develops a growth problem and is growing at a very slow rate but has not yet dropped outside the normal range. To understand when a child's growth pattern is worrisome, we need to look beyond the simple statistical definition of *normal*. We need to consider several factors.

Height Percentile

First, we need to consider the child's height percentile. This tells us whether the current height is within the normal range or not.

Family Background

A second factor to consider is the height of close family members, especially parents but also siblings and to a lesser degree grandparents. If a child is at the 3rd percentile and both parents are also at the 3rd percentile, we are not as concerned as we would be if the child was at the 3rd percentile and the parents were at the 75th. That's common sense.

Often we find that a short but healthy child is brought to see a growth specialist because a younger sibling or cousin is noted to be catching up in height. To a child, it may seem terribly unfair that a younger sibling is catching up and in some cases overtaking him or her. When this occurs, it's worth bringing the situation to the attention of the child's pediatrician. There are indeed cases in which this discrepancy is a clue to an abnormal slowing of growth in the older child. Still, in most such cases, the growth chart shows that the short child is growing steadily near the low end of the normal range, and an evaluation reveals that the child is healthy. As noted in chapter 2, there can be a great deal of variability within a family in the heights and growth rates of individual children, and the most common explanation is that the younger sibling or cousin has inherited genes that allow for more rapid growth.

Growth Rate

A third factor to consider is the child's growth rate—how fast he or she is growing. If we had two heights measured a year apart, we could calculate the growth rate in inches per year. However, this sort of calculation is often misleading, especially if the heights were not done on a stadiometer by an experienced person. Alternatively, we can try to judge the growth rate by looking at the recent portion of the child's growth curve. Hopefully there will be several points on the curve within the past couple of years, and we can judge how the child's growth curve compares with normal percentile curves. This comparison, illustrated by the growth chart in figure 4, is helpful in assessing growth. If the child is growing parallel to a normal percentile curve (curve A), it suggests that the child's growth rate is normal. If the child's growth curve is cutting across the normal percentile curves, shifting to lower percentiles over time (curve B), it suggests that the growth rate is abnormally

CDC Growth Charts: United States

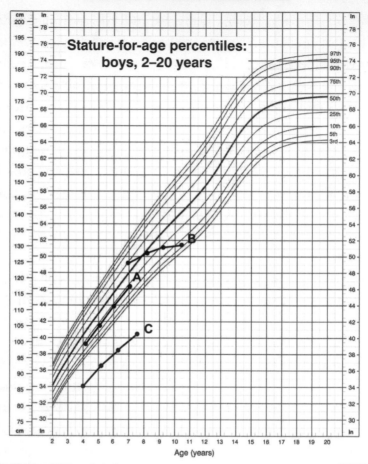

Stature-for-age percentiles: boys, 2–20 years

Modified from NCHS growth charts:
Published May 30, 2000.
SOURCE: Developed by the National Center for Health Statistics in collaboration with
the National Center for Chronic Disease Prevention and Health Promotion (2000).

CDC
SAFER · HEALTHIER · PEOPLE™

Figure 4. Different patterns of growth. The growth chart is for boys age 2–20 years. Curve A represents a boy whose height is tracking parallel to, and just below, the 25th percentile curve. He has a normal growth rate. Curve B represents a boy whose height was initially at the 75th percentile but over time dropped to the 5th. This boy has an abnormally low growth rate. Curve C represents a boy who initially is well below the 3rd percentile and over time is gradually falling farther from the normal range. His growth rate is also slightly decreased.

58

low. This pattern is more worrisome. Even though the child's current height is still normal, the low growth rate raises the concern that some recent problem might be interfering with growth. A third growth pattern is shown in curve C. This child is falling farther and farther away from the 3rd percentile. In this case, the child's current height is abnormal and his growth rate is also probably abnormal. This pattern is also worrisome.

We can also make the same sort of assessment of the child's weight gain. Is the weight gain paralleling the normal percentile curves or is it cutting across the normal percentile curves, shifting to lower percentiles, or falling farther and farther from the 3rd percentile? The same principle that we discussed for height applies here: If a child's weight curve is not paralleling the normal percentile curves, the level of concern is raised.

To be honest, we've oversimplified things. In real life, the growth data, especially the height data, are rarely so precise and smooth. They bounce up and down because, as we discussed, kids are hard to measure accurately. So we are often unsure: Is the child growing poorly or do we just have inaccurate measurements? This imprecision is one reason why it takes experience to read a growth chart well.

We are frequently asked to see children who have for several years been growing steadily along one of the percentile curves at the lower part of the normal range, and at one visit the height seems to have increased very little since the previous measurement 6 to 12 months ago, causing a "bend" in the growth curve. In most of these cases, the child has experienced no change in health. We find that slowing of growth based on a single point is more often due to measurement error than to actual medical problems. In this situation, the first step in the evaluation should be to make additional careful measurements before you leave the doctor's office that day to see whether they confirm the slowing in growth.

Comparing Height and Weight Percentiles

When evaluating a child's growth chart, a fourth factor to consider is the weight percentile and how it compares with the height percentile. If a child's height is at the 3rd percentile but her weight is well below the 3rd percentile, she probably looks skinny, and we might wonder if there is some problem with nutrition or food absorption. On the other hand, if her weight is at the 3rd percentile and her height is well below this percentile, it makes us think of certain endocrine diseases. Again, we've oversimplified matters to get the concept across. In real life, there are many diagnoses to consider; the relationship between height and weight does not usually let us absolutely rule in or out any specific diagnoses. But it is another useful clue, a piece of the puzzle.

Health

A fifth factor to consider is the child's health. Is he completely healthy or are there some health concerns? Even if he just has one or more isolated symptoms, we should think about whether they could be related to his growth pattern. For example, if your child is small for his age and has problems with diarrhea or abdominal pain, we might think about certain GI disorders. On the other hand, if he has been growing poorly for the last year or two and is having severe or increasingly frequent headaches, we should think about problems in the pituitary or nearby areas of the brain.

WHEN DOES SHORT STATURE NEED TO BE EVALUATED BY A PHYSICIAN?

Of course, all children should be visiting their pediatrician, family doctor, or other health professional for regular health care. At these regular checkups, the provider should measure the height and weight and plot the values on a growth chart. If the provider sees an abnormal pattern, he or she should discuss this with you. And if you are concerned about your child's growth, you should bring up the subject, even if your health care provider doesn't. So when should you be concerned? Let's go through some examples.

- **Your child's height and weight are tracking along the 25th percentile** (see curve A in figure 5). If you and your spouse are on the short side, there's usually no need for worry. True, your child is shorter than average (the 50th percentile), but he or she is still within the normal range (between the 3rd and 97th percentiles). Someone has to be shorter than average.

CDC Growth Charts: United States

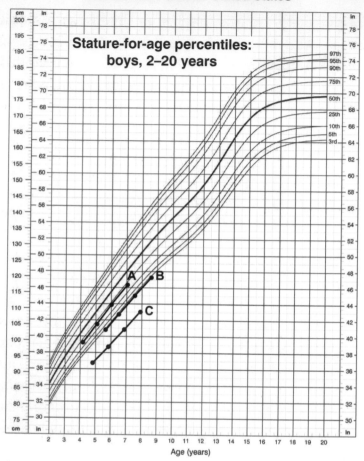

Stature-for-age percentiles: boys, 2–20 years

Modified from NCHS growth charts:
Published May 30, 2000.
SOURCE: Developed by the National Center for Health Statistics in collaboration with
the National Center for Chronic Disease Prevention and Health Promotion (2000).

Figure 5. Different patterns of growth. The growth chart is for boys age 2–20 years. Curve A represents a boy whose height is tracking parallel to, and just below, the 25th percentile curve. Curve B represents a boy whose height is tracking parallel to, and just below, the 3rd percentile. Curve C represents a boy who is growing parallel to, but well below, the 3rd percentile.

- **Your child's height and weight are tracking along or just below the 3rd percentile** (see curve B in figure 5). If you and your spouse are short, your child may just have inherited genes for shortness from you. However, you should bring the growth pattern to the attention of your doctor at the time of checkups and ask for his or her thoughts. Ask whether the doctor thinks your child's growth is appropriate for the family background. If your child has this growth pattern but you and your spouse are of average height or on the tall side, the level of concern would be greater.

- **Your child's height or weight is well below the 3rd percentile** (see curve C in figure 5). You should definitely discuss the growth pattern with a health care provider.

- **Your child's height and/or weight is still within the normal range but is crossing percentiles downward over time** (see curve D in figure 6). You should discuss the growth pattern with a health care provider. For example, a child who had been growing along the 75th percentile and then over time shifted to the 10th percentile may have a problem interfering with growth.

- **Your child's height is below the 3rd percentile and over time is falling farther from the normal range** (see curve E in figure 6). Both your child's current height and his or her growth rate are decreased. This also is a worrisome growth pattern.

As we discussed above, if a child is experiencing other health problems, then the level of concern is increased. On

CDC Growth Charts: United States

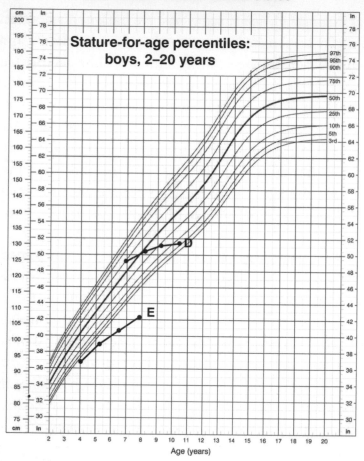

Stature-for-age percentiles:
boys, 2–20 years

Modified from NCHS growth charts:
Published May 30, 2000.
SOURCE: Developed by the National Center for Health Statistics in collaboration with
the National Center for Chronic Disease Prevention and Health Promotion (2000).

Figure 6. Different patterns of growth. The growth chart is for boys age 2–20 years. Curve D represents a boy whose height is initially at the 75th percentile but over time dropped to the 5th. We say that he is crossing percentiles. He has an abnormally low growth rate. This is a worrisome growth pattern. Curve E represents a boy whose height is below the 3rd percentile and over time is falling farther from the normal range. His current height and his growth rate are both decreased. This also is a worrisome growth pattern.

the other hand, the absence of other symptoms does not exclude the possibility that there might be an underlying health problem. Sometimes health problems can show up first in the growth chart.

The bottom line is this: When in doubt, talk to your child's health care provider. That's what providers are there for.

KEY POINTS TO KEEP IN MIND

Measuring height accurately is not easy. Even a careful measurement has some uncertainty. Children's height and weight measurements should be plotted on growth charts. From the growth chart, we determine the child's height percentile—how his or her height compares with children the same age. However, to evaluate a child's growth, we also need to consider other factors, including the height of family members, the child's growth rate, how the height and weight percentile compare, and the child's health. Evaluating these factors requires experience, which is one reason you should bring your child to the pediatrician for regular health care visits. In addition, if you notice that your child has an abnormal height or weight, or an abnormal growth rate in height or weight, discuss your child's growth with the pediatrician.

CHAPTER 6

Predicting Adult Height

Prediction is very difficult, especially about the future.
—NIELS BOHR

In the last chapter, we addressed the question, *Is my child's height normal?* Here we try to tackle a question that is even more difficult: *Will my child's height be normal when he or she is fully grown?* Many parents are deeply concerned that their child will not attain a normal adult size. Others are just curious about how tall their child will be when fully grown. Although we cannot provide a crystal ball, we can discuss some of the important concepts related to height prediction.

PREDICTION METHODS

It would be useful to have a precise method to predict the adult height of a child accurately. It would allay unnecessary worry and help parents and physicians decide when to consider a medical intervention. Unfortunately, there are no precise methods to do so—only approximate methods.

Some are better than others, but they are still just educated guesses. The bottom line is that even the best methods can be wrong.

Target Height

In chapter 2, we discussed the target height, which is an adjusted average of the parents' heights. If you look at large groups of children, this method has some validity. On average, children tend to end up somewhat close to their parents' heights. But as we also noted in chapter 2, there is a lot of variability. A child may have inherited the "taller genes" or the "shorter genes" from his or her parents. So for the individual child, this method is not a great predictor. Kids just don't always end up the same height as their parents, even if they are completely healthy. If they are ill, this throws another complicating variable into the prediction.

Birth Size

Some methods used to predict adult height are quite inaccurate. For example, you cannot predict adult height accurately based on a child's birth size, which is affected by conditions in the uterus. Following birth, the child's situation changes and the growth pattern can shift. The biggest shifts occur in the first 18 months of age. A child who was born large for his or her gestational age—let's say at the 95th percentile—may shift percentiles downward during the first 12 to 18 months and then track along a lower percentile, perhaps the 50th. Conversely, a child who is born small for gestational age—say, at the 5th percentile—may catch up during the first couple of years of life and then track along the 50th percentile.

Doubling the Height at Age Two

You may have heard that you can predict your child's adult height by taking the height at two years of age and doubling it. This method, too, is inaccurate. On average, it will overestimate the adult height in girls and underestimate it in boys. And for any individual child, we can't even make this generalization.

Following the Child's Percentile on the Growth Chart

Another way to predict height is to plot the child's height on the growth chart and note which percentile it falls on. Then you can follow that percentile curve up and to the right until it levels off and then read the height at which the curve hits the Y-axis. This method might be better than the first two, but it still isn't particularly good. It assumes that a child at the 5th percentile, for example, will remain at the 5th percentile. It is true that most healthy children will grow pretty much along a percentile curve between about 2 years old and about 10 or 12. However, children often shift percentiles around the time of puberty. If healthy children experience puberty on the late side, they tend to end up at a higher percentile as adults than they followed in childhood. If they hit puberty on the early side, they tend to end up at a lower percentile. The problem with this method, then, is that it doesn't take into account the child's tempo of maturation (see chapter 1). In addition, some children have a greater growth spurt during puberty than others, and this may also cause a shift in growth percentile.

Bone Age Methods

A child's bone age is assessed by taking an X-ray of the left hand and wrist. An experienced physician can use this X-ray to see how mature the bones appear. In a young child, the bones contain areas made of cartilage. As the child gets older, most of that cartilage gets changed into actual bone tissue. The X-ray reveals how far along the child has progressed in this maturational process. The reading physician will compare it with an atlas showing X-rays of normal children. If the patient's X-ray most closely matches that of an average 6-year-old child, we say that the patient has a bone age of 6 years.

Children with a slow tempo of maturation tend to have a delayed bone age. For a slowly maturing 9-year-old child, the bone age might be 7 years. Conversely, children with a rapid tempo of maturation tend to have an advanced bone age. So a rapidly maturing 9-year-old child might have a bone age of 11 years.

The bone age helps us estimate how much growth capacity remains in the growth plates. On average, that 9-year-old with a bone age of 7 years will have more growth in his or her future than the 9-year-old with a bone age of 11. To make the height prediction, the physician takes the child's current height and bone age and then uses mathematical tables to find the predicted adult height. The tables begin at approximately 6 years of age, so we cannot use this method to predict the height of a younger child.

The bone age method of prediction is the best readily available method. But it is still not highly accurate for several reasons. First, reading a bone age is not like doing a laboratory test; it is more subjective. The interpretation is usually done by a radiologist (X-ray specialist) or pediatric endocrinologist. It requires experience, and it requires the patience to look at many individual bones carefully. For this reason, we tend to read the bone age X-rays of our patients ourselves, unless they were read by someone whom we know and trust. When we review bone age X-rays, we often find that they had previously been misread. Even two careful, skilled observers won't agree exactly. Because bone ages are often read inaccurately, it may not be a good idea for a primary care physician to order one unless he or she knows that the radiologist reading it is particularly skilled in this assessment.

A second problem with the method is that the tables used for height prediction are based on normal, not short, children. If your child has an illness, the prediction may not be accurate. Even in children with delayed maturation or familial short stature, this prediction method has some problems.

A third problem is that each child is unique. The human body is very complicated, and simple rules cannot capture all the complexity.

As a result of all these issues, height prediction with a bone age is only a rough estimate. Even in healthy children of normal height—who don't really need a height prediction—it is not unusual for children to end up with an adult height that is 2 inches more or less than the predicted height. For children with short stature, this error may be even greater.

In general, the older the child, the more accurate the prediction. It's like archery: The closer you stand to the target, the easier it is to hit the bull's-eye. Or to put it another way, if you are driving from the East Coast to the West Coast, the prediction of your arrival time that you make as you enter California will be far more accurate than the one made as you crossed the Mississippi. So our height prediction for a 13-year-old child tends to be more accurate than our prediction for a 7-year-old.

Why even bother to do a height prediction based on bone age? Families want to know what to expect for their child, and this is the best method we have. It can be somewhat helpful, but we keep in mind the possible error. Unfortunately, it's hard to really understand the uncertainty. We like to think that a statement is either right or wrong, not in between. Sometimes we hear a parent say something like, "The doctor predicted that my daughter would end up 4 feet, 11 inches, but he was wrong. She only ended up 4 feet, 10 inches." Either the doctor did not explain the uncertainty of height prediction, or perhaps the parents—overloaded with too much information in the clinic that day—did not understand or forgot the uncertainty.

Often it's better to think of the height prediction not as a single number, but as a range. If the height prediction is 5 feet, 6 inches, the doctor might say that 5 feet, 6 inches, is the best guess, and that the child will probably end up somewhere between 5 feet, 4 inches, and 5 feet, 8 inches. The width of the range depends on the individual circumstances, including the age; a wider range will usually be given for a younger child than an older. Even when we provide a range, we have to admit that it's not guaranteed. It is possible that the child will end up even farther from the height prediction.

The analogy to archery is useful to keep in mind. Occasionally the arrow hits the bull's-eye. Usually it hits the target somewhere. Once in a while, it misses completely.

PREDICTING HEIGHT IN CHILDREN WITH CHRONIC ILLNESS

If a child has an illness that is interfering with growth, then height prediction is even more difficult. Remember that the height prediction tables are based on the growth of normal children. Besides, how could a table "know" whether a child's illness will worsen, stay the same, or improve? Still, there is a concept that helps us a bit. It's known as catch-up growth.

Catch-Up Growth

Suppose a child has an illness that is interfering with her growth—say, hypothyroidism. By the time the illness is discovered, she may be quite short (see figure 7). Suppose also that either the disease resolves on its own, or, in the case of hypothyroidism, there is a good treatment for it. When the child is restored to health, we might expect her growth rate to return to normal. If that happened, she would stay short. Her height would remain below the normal range and her growth curve would be parallel to, but below, the 3rd percentile. However, this usually does not happen. Instead, when health is restored, the growth rate often does not just return to normal but actually exceeds normal. The child's height climbs back up toward the normal range, or even into the normal range (as in figure 7). This phenomenon, catch-up growth, can occur after a wide variety of growth-inhibiting conditions, including hypothyroidism, Cushing syndrome, growth hormone deficiency, malnutrition, and many chronic diseases. However, strong catch-up growth usually occurs only if the underlying health problem resolves (or greatly improves) either on its own or with treatment.

Unfortunately, catch-up growth is often not complete. In other words, the child's height percentile climbs back up toward normal but may not reach the normal range. Or it may reach the normal range but not the height percentile that the child would have been on had there been no problem. As in all matters of pediatric medicine, we must remember that each child is different.

Some of the catch-up growth occurs over the first couple of years after the illness resolves. In addition, the illness may slow the child's tempo of maturation, and so the re-

CDC Growth Charts: United States

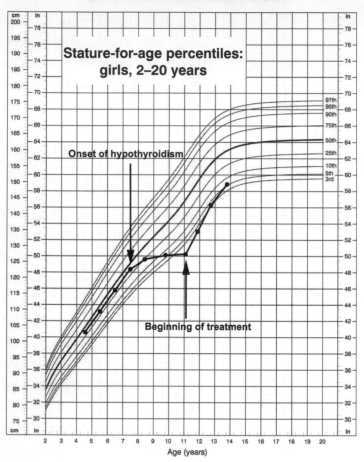

Stature-for-age percentiles: girls, 2–20 years

Onset of hypothyroidism

Beginning of treatment

Age (years)

Modified from NCHS growth charts:
Published May 30, 2000.
SOURCE: Developed by the National Center for Health Statistics in collaboration with
the National Center for Chronic Disease Prevention and Health Promotion (2000).

Figure 7. Growth chart of a girl with hypothyroidism, showing catch-up growth after treatment. This girl developed hypothyroidism at approximately age eight. Afterward, her growth rate was very poor until 11 years of age, when the problem was detected and she started to take thyroid hormone medication. Her growth rate didn't just normalize but actually became greater than normal—catch-up growth.

covered child may have a late puberty and keep growing longer than other children. Often a bone age will help tell us whether the illness slowed down the child's tempo of maturation. However, in this setting we should rely even less on the exact bone-age-based height prediction than usual.

KEY POINTS TO KEEP IN MIND

It is difficult to predict a child's adult height. Part of the reason is that children often cross percentiles around the time of puberty. The best readily available method is the bone age X-ray, yet this method has serious limitations. The bone age must be read by someone with experience and diligence, and even so the prediction is only approximate. In children who are ill, prediction is even more difficult. If the illness resolves or is effectively treated, the child will often experience some catch-up growth, although it may not be complete.

CHAPTER 7

The Many Causes of Short Stature

Up to now, our focus has been on normal growth. We have discussed the factors that regulate growth, how to determine whether a child's growth is normal, and the methods we use for predicting adult height. We have focused on normal growth because most short children do not have an important underlying illness. They are healthy children who happen to be short. Many come from short families. Some are just slow maturers who will end up at a normal height as adults. However, a minority of short children are short because of some underlying medical disorder. Of those with a true medical diagnosis, only a small proportion are actually short due to insufficient growth hormone. Some may have an obvious illness, but other children have poor growth because of a subtle, unrecognized medical problem.

In this chapter, we will outline the major causes of short stature that physicians need to consider, starting with the two most common diagnoses, constitutional growth delay and familial short stature. In both conditions, the child is healthy but short. We will then proceed to specific medical conditions. The list of diagnoses we will cover is given in table 6. This is not meant to be an exhaustive list of all possible causes—which would be very long indeed. Instead the table, and this chapter in general, focuses on some of the more common causes of short stature. Our aim is to give you an idea of the large number of different problems that can impair growth.

Table 6. Major Causes of Short Stature

Normal variant growth patterns
    Constitutional growth delay
    Familial short stature
    Combination of the two
Chromosomal abnormalities
    Turner syndrome
    Down syndrome
Skeletal dysplasias (abnormalities of bone formation)
Other genetic syndromes
    Russell-Silver syndrome
    Noonan syndrome
    Prader-Willi syndrome
Intrauterine growth retardation without a specific syndrome
Endocrine disorders
    Hypothyroidism
    Cushing syndrome
    Early puberty

> Poorly controlled diabetes
> Growth hormone deficiency
> Undernutrition
> Chronic disease
> Chronic gastrointestinal disorders
> Inflammatory bowel disease
> Celiac disease
> Kidney disorders
> Chronic renal failure
> Renal tubular acidosis
> Other chronic diseases
> Medications
> Corticosteroids
> Stimulant medications (used for attention deficit disorder)
> Idiopathic short stature (unknown cause)

NORMAL VARIANT GROWTH PATTERNS

Constitutional Growth Delay

Constitutional growth delay is a common cause of short stature in childhood. It is, in essence, the medical term for a child who is healthy but tends to mature slowly. The word *constitutional* is an old term meaning that the condition is part of the person's nature and does not come from some outside problem. In this condition, the child's biological clock is ticking more slowly than normal; he or she typically grows slowly, goes through puberty late, keeps growing till a later age than usual, and often (but not always) ends up at a normal height.

For reasons that are not clear, the diagnosis of constitutional growth delay is more common in boys than girls.

The growth pattern associated with this diagnosis is very characteristic. Typically, these children have a normal birth weight, but then, between six months and about two years of age, growth is a bit slower than average so that height and weight dip to below the 5th percentile. After age two to three years, the rate of growth normalizes, so that the child's height and usually weight as well are tracking a little below but parallel to the 5th percentile curve (see figure 8). This trend continues through most of childhood until the time when normal girls and boys start their adolescent growth spurts, which is around 11 or 12 years in girls and 13 to 14 in boys. At this time, children with constitutional growth delay fall farther behind their peers, because their adolescent growth spurt is delayed. However, about the time that normal children are finishing their growth spurts, children with constitutional growth delay start theirs, and by the time they are 15 to 16 (girls) or 17 to 18 (boys), they have often caught up to the normal range in height—usually the lower half of the normal range.

How can we tell that a short child most likely has constitutional growth delay? First of all, the growth pattern described above is typical. In these children, review of the growth records shows that they have been growing parallel to, but slightly below, the 5th percentile since they were toddlers. Second, this condition often runs in families; in

CDC Growth Charts: United States

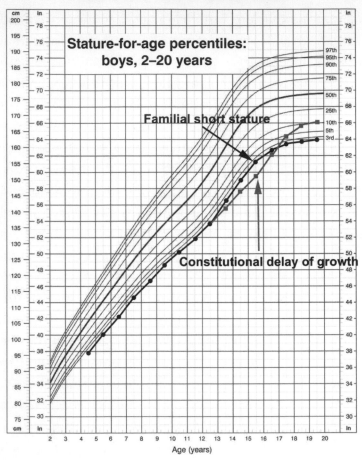

Stature-for-age percentiles: boys, 2–20 years

Familial short stature

Constitutional delay of growth

Age (years)

Modified from NCHS growth charts:
Published May 30, 2000.
SOURCE: Developed by the National Center for Health Statistics in collaboration with
the National Center for Chronic Disease Prevention and Health Promotion (2000).

CDC
SAFER · HEALTHIER · PEOPLE™

Figure 8. Growth chart of a boy with familial short stature and one with constitutional delay of growth. Initially, the two curves are the same; both boys are growing parallel to, and just below, the 3rd percentile. However, the boy with familial short stature remains below the 3rd percentile during adolescence and ends up short as an adult. The boy with constitutional delay actually falls farther behind normal children during adolescence because he has a delayed growth spurt. However, he catches up later when he eventually has his growth spurt and then continues to grow later than most boys. These curves are just examples; every child is different. Many children appear to have a mixture of familial short stature and constitutional delay.

many cases, one of the parents or another family member had a similar growth pattern as well as a late puberty. For example, the mother may tell us that she started her periods later than normal (after age 14), or the father had his growth spurt later than normal and was still growing (or had just stopped growing) at the time he graduated from high school. Both of these situations suggest delayed onset of puberty. Third, after taking a careful medical history, doing a careful physical exam, and, if necessary, performing some screening laboratory tests, we can find no evidence of an underlying illness. Fourth, we can obtain an X-ray of the hand for a bone age, which is usually delayed by two or more years in children with constitutional growth delay. Just as other aspects of physical maturation are delayed, the maturation of the bones is also delayed so that a typical 10-year-old child with constitutional growth delay might have an X-ray that looks like that of an average 8-year-old. In this case we would say that the bone age was delayed by two years. However, a delayed bone age is not by itself diagnostic of constitutional growth delay; many other conditions also delay bone age. As discussed in chapter 6, the bone age can be used to predict adult height, and typically children with constitutional growth delay have a height prediction in the low-normal range. Although some children, particularly boys, may not quite reach their predicted height, this information can be reassuring to parents who are worried that their child has been growing consistently below the normal range, and is one reason for not recommending growth hormone treatment for these children, unless their predicted height is well below the normal range.

Familial Short Stature

A second common cause of short stature is familial short stature. Like children with constitutional growth delay, these children are often referred to specialists in mid-childhood and are growing at a normal rate, parallel to but at or a little below the 5th percentile curve (see figure 8). The difference is that, unlike those with constitutional growth delay, children with familial short stature have one or two short parents (hence the term *familial*), and their bone age is usually within a year of their actual age. In classic familial short stature, the height we predict, based on the bone age, is often below the normal range (less than 5 feet, 5 inches, for boys, or less than 5 feet for girls) but usually within 2 inches of the target height based on the parents' height (see chapter 2). Typically, children with familial short stature will end up short as adults, like their parents.

Although many short children we see fit neatly into one of these two categories, there are many who seem to have a combination of constitutional growth delay and familial short stature. For example, we may be evaluating a short boy whose parents are also somewhat short but who has a bone age delayed by two or more years as well. In such cases, we may tell the parents that their son is still a short healthy child, but he has features suggesting a combination of factors affecting his growth. Due to the delay in bone age, such a child may end up less short than you'd expect solely from looking at his growth chart: His delayed bone age predicts a late puberty and additional time to grow before his growth plates fuse.

CHROMOSOMAL ABNORMALITIES

As discussed in chapter 2, children can be short if they do not have a normal number of chromosomes. We will only discuss two of the more common chromosomal abnormalities, Turner syndrome and Down syndrome.

Turner Syndrome

Turner syndrome affects about 1 in 2,500 girls and is caused by a missing X chromosome (or a missing part of the X chromosome). Recall that normal boys have one X and one Y chromosome, whereas normal girls have two X chromosomes. Girls with Turner syndrome typically have only one X chromosome and no Y.

At birth, these girls tend to be low-normal in weight (average birth weight 6 pounds, 3 ounces). Their growth in length usually starts to drop below the normal range between one and two years of age, and they usually continue to fall farther behind with time. Growth charts specific for Turner syndrome are available.

In girls with this syndrome, the ovaries usually do not function normally. As a result, these girls may not show signs of puberty, especially breast development, or they may have some puberty before the ovaries fail. The lack of estrogens resulting from this ovarian failure can be corrected by providing estrogen medication, usually starting at age 12 to 15.

A diagnosis of Turner syndrome is sometimes suspected in the newborn period based on swelling of the hands and feet due to lymphedema (poor lymph drainage), which resolves over time. In older girls, the diagnosis may be suspected in an individual with short stature and/or delayed puberty. Often, these girls have certain other physical features that help point toward the diagnosis, including extra skin folds causing a wide neck (seen in 40 percent of girls with Turner syndrome); a high-arched and narrow palate, or roof of the mouth (75 percent); low-set ears (60 percent); arms bent slightly outward at the elbows when the palms face forward (50 percent); short knuckles of the fourth finger (33 percent); and fingernails and toenails that angle upward (75 percent).

Confirming the diagnosis requires analysis of the chromosomes (called a karyotype) in a genetics laboratory, a test that can be done on a blood sample. Some girls, particularly those who are missing only part of an X chromosome or who are missing all or part of the X chromosome in only some of their cells (we call this mosaicism), may look completely normal except for being short. Therefore, a karyotype is often done in any girl who has significant, unexplained short stature.

Without treatment of their short stature, the average adult height of patients with Turner syndrome in the United States is about 4 feet, 8 or 9 inches, but can vary widely in different individuals. As discussed later, the use of growth hormone can add several inches to these girls' height.

Girls and women with Turner syndrome have a higher risk for certain medical problems, including congenital heart disease, kidney abnormalities, frequent ear infections, high blood pressure, and hypothyroidism. These girls should therefore be carefully evaluated and followed by a physician who is knowledgeable about this condition. Parents wishing to learn more about Turner syndrome can go to the Web site of the Turner Syndrome Society (www .turner-syndrome-us.org).

Down Syndrome

Down syndrome is a common condition that occurs when a child has three copies of chromosome 21 instead of the normal two copies. Its frequency is about 1 in 1,000 births. Increased maternal age is a risk factor. These children can be diagnosed based on their characteristic facial appearance and other physical signs, followed by a karyotype. Down syndrome usually affects intelligence and can be associated with certain birth defects. Children with Down syndrome are usually shorter than their peers. The average height of adult males is about 4 feet, 11 inches; for adult females, about 4 feet, 8 inches. Special growth charts have been produced for tracking the growth of these children. In contrast with Turner syndrome, most physicians are not currently recommending growth hormone treatment in Down syndrome. Children with Down syndrome are at increased risk for certain medical problems and should be followed by a physician knowledgeable about this disorder.

SKELETAL DYSPLASIAS

A skeletal dysplasia is a disorder in which the child's bones have an abnormal shape and size because of a genetic abnormality. There are many different skeletal dsyplasias due to mutations in different genes. Some affect the bones in the spine more, while others affect the bones in the arms and legs. As a result, many skeletal dysplasias are characterized by disproportionate growth. For example, the legs and arms may be short but the trunk and head may be unaffected. A quick (but imperfect) test for this disproportion is to have children stand with their hands at their sides and see where the tips of their fingers touch their sides. In people with normal proportions, the fingertips usually reach to the middle of their thighs, while in people with short arms, the fingertips may reach only the upper thighs or hips. Another way to check for abnormal proportions is to measure the arm span. The child is asked to stand with arms outstretched, and the distance from fingertip to fingertip is measured and compared with the child's height. In normal children, the arm span is similar to the height, while in skeletal dysplasias that affect the limbs more than the spine, the arm span will be significantly less than the height. X-rays are also used to detect the bone abnormalities in this condition.

The most common type of skeletal dysplasia is called

achondroplasia, which has an incidence of 1 in 15,000–
40,000. The average height of adults with achondroplasia
is about 4 feet, 1 inch, for females and 4 feet, 4 inches, for
males. Since the arms and legs are unusually short, by
comparison, the trunk and head appear relatively large.
This condition can be inherited as a dominant trait—if a
parent is affected, there is a 50 percent chance that his or
her children will be affected. However, the majority of
children with achondroplasia are born to two unaffected
parents because of a new mutation in the child's DNA, in
a gene coding for the protein FGF receptor-3. The diagnosis can be made based on the physical appearance and
the abnormal shape of the long bones on an X-ray or
genetic test. Growth hormone has been tried in achondroplasia, but the result has been only a slight improvement in growth. Orthopedic surgery has also been used to
lengthen the patient's legs. The long bones in the legs are
broken; a metal device is then attached to the bone to
slowly separate the two ends as they heal. As you might
imagine, there are major drawbacks to this approach.

A milder form of skeletal dysplasia, hypochondroplasia, is due to a less severe mutation of the FGF receptor-3
gene. Like achondroplasia, hypochondroplasia affects the
growth of the long bones more than the spine.

There are many other skeletal dysplasias, some that
affect primarily long bones and others that affect mainly
the bones of the spine. These conditions are best diagnosed by a specialist in genetics, who can order a series of
X-rays to reveal the bone abnormalities characteristic of

these conditions. With time, the number of disorders that can be detected with a genetic test on a blood sample is increasing.

OTHER GENETIC SYNDROMES ASSOCIATED WITH SHORT STATURE

There are a large number of conditions, most of them rare, in which a short child also exhibits certain other characteristic abnormalities. Many children with these genetic syndromes have a distinctive appearance. The diagnosis is often based on the combination of abnormalities. In some disorders, it can be confirmed by a specific laboratory test. Geneticists are the specialists most experienced at diagnosing these syndromes.

Although the diagnosis of a specific syndrome does not by itself help a child grow taller, it will help alert the parents and the physicians to specific physical and learning problems the child may have or develop. While most of these syndromes are so rare that it would not be helpful in a book of this type to describe all of their characteristic features, we will describe three genetic syndromes that are relatively common and serve as good examples of this general category.

Russell-Silver Syndrome

Russell-Silver syndrome is one of the more common genetic syndromes that cause short stature (incidence about 1 in 3,000 children). These children are typically already small at birth—about 4 to 5 pounds for a full-term child. The most common physical feature is a face of triangular shape, with a broad forehead, a small narrow chin, and downturned corners of the mouth. About half of these children will have asymmetry of the limbs, meaning that one arm or leg will be shorter than the other. In many children the little finger is curved. Intelligence is typically normal. Untreated, the average adult height is about 5 feet for males and 4 feet, 7 inches, for females.

Noonan Syndrome

This syndrome is characterized by short stature, extra skin folds causing a wide neck, arms bent slightly outward at the elbows, and congenital heart disease (features similar to those of Turner syndrome). Distinctive facial features may include low-set ears, flattening of the upper nose, and eyes set far apart with drooping eyelids. The frequency of Noonan syndrome is about 1 in 2,000 children. Puberty is delayed, and adult height is often at the low end of the normal range.

Prader-Willi Syndrome

The major features of Prader-Willi syndrome include severe obesity starting between ages one and six, uncontrolled appetite, mild to moderate short stature, mental retardation, and small genitalia. One useful clue is a history of decreased movement when the child was still in the womb, and poor muscle tone ("floppiness") in infancy. This syndrome occurs in about 1 in 20,000 individuals, and the diagnosis can sometimes be confirmed by a genetic test on a blood sample.

INTRAUTERINE GROWTH RETARDATION

Sometimes a child grows poorly before birth. This condition is referred to as intrauterine growth retardation (*intrauterine* indicates that it occurred while the child was within the uterus). When this occurs, the child is born small for gestational age, meaning that his or her birth size is decreased for the length of the pregnancy. In other words, the child is small at birth, and the decreased size is not just due to prematurity.

Sometimes, the reason for the intrauterine growth retardation is evident—for example, in children with Russell-Silver syndrome (see above)—but often there are no other findings suggesting a specific syndrome or disease. In some children, intrauterine growth retardation may occur because placental function was not sufficient for optimal growth, but it is often hard to be sure of the cause in an individual child.

In most such cases, children born small for gestational age will catch up into the normal range by two years of age. For instance, if one of a pair of twins was small at birth due to crowding in the womb, he or she will often be back on the normal growth curve by age one or two. However, about 10 percent of children born small for gestational age fail to catch up by age two. In the past decade, research studies have demonstrated that growth hormone treatment will increase growth in these children.

ENDOCRINE DISORDERS

Endocrine (hormone-related) disorders were introduced in chapter 4 in our discussion of the general effects of hormones on growth. Here, we will focus on the diagnosis and treatment of specific endocrine disorders that cause short stature.

One clue that an endocrine problem may be causing short stature is that the height is often affected by the disorder more than the weight. In other words, children with endocrine disorders may experience slow gain in height while continuing to gain weight more normally or even rapidly. As a result, kids with endocrine disorders usually do not appear to be skinny and may even appear overweight. In contrast, children with undernutrition and chronic illness usually do appear thin because their weight gain is more affected than their height gain. Of course, there are exceptions to these rules.

Hypothyroidism

As discussed in chapter 4, thyroid hormone is required for normal growth during childhood. Hypothyroidism that is present from birth, called congenital hypothyroidism, is usually detected in the first weeks of life by newborn screening tests and treated before there is any detectable effect on growth. However, hypothyroidism that begins sometime after birth, or acquired hypothyroidism, often causes short stature. If the hypothyroidism is severe enough and remains undetected for long enough, it can slow growth in height almost to a standstill. Acquired hypothyroidism is most often due to a gradual, painless destruction of the thyroid gland by the body's immune system. This condition is called autoimmune thyroiditis or Hashimoto's thyroiditis. In many cases, there is an increase in the size of the thyroid gland, which can lead to diagnosis and treatment before severe growth failure occurs. In other cases, there is little thyroid enlargement or the enlargement goes unnoticed; the condition may not be detected until long after its onset, resulting in more severe growth failure.

Symptoms that suggest this diagnosis include fatigue, dry skin, constipation, feeling cold when others are comfortable, and decreased appetite. However, not all hypothyroid individuals will have all these symptoms. In fact, some children with hypothyroidism will have poor growth but few other symptoms. Therefore, most physicians will do a blood test for hypothyroidism in any child with significant, unexplained short stature.

The blood tests for hypothyroidism are commonly called thyroid function tests. Diagnosis of hypothyroidism is easily made if the blood level of thyroid hormone is low and the level of thyroid-stimulating hormone (TSH) is very high. This elevated level of TSH represents the pituitary gland's attempt to correct the low level of thyroid hormone. However, we are often asked to see children who have normal levels of thyroid hormone, only a minimal elevation of TSH, and no antibodies in the blood to suggest autoimmune thyroiditis; in this common situation, it is not clear that a thyroid problem is slowing growth, and some endocrinologists will not treat with thyroid hormone but just have the thyroid tests rechecked periodically. Children found to have clear-cut hypothyroidism are treated with thyroid hormone tablets and usually undergo at least partial catch-up growth (see figure 7).

Cushing Syndrome

This condition can result either from overproduction of the hormone cortisol by the adrenal glands or from taking corticosteroid medication (see chapter 4). Onset can be at any age, and the growth chart will usually show height crossing percentiles downward while weight crosses percentiles upward. The child usually looks overweight. The face often develops a round appearance. Purple stretch marks can occur. If it's not caused by corticosteroid medication, Cushing syndrome is usually attributable to either a tumor of the adrenal glands, which overproduces cortisol, or a tumor of the pituitary gland, which produces an adrenal-stimulating hormone called ACTH. Once the exact cause is identified, the best treatment is usually surgery to remove the adrenal or pituitary tumor. However, the proper diagnosis and treatment of Cushing syndrome can sometimes be difficult and may require referral to a medical center with expertise in this rare disorder.

Early Puberty

Endocrinologists are often asked to evaluate teenagers whose growth has slowed or stopped at an age when most other children are still growing. This often occurs because puberty started a couple of years earlier than average and the child is already late in puberty (see figure 9). If a short teenage girl is already having menstrual periods, or if a teenage boy is in late puberty, the child's growth is usually starting to taper off. In some cases, the growth plates may already have disappeared. Once the growth plates disappear or have nearly disappeared, treatment with growth hormone or other medications will not produce significant additional growth.

Poorly Controlled Diabetes

Children with well-controlled diabetes generally grow well. If the diabetes is poorly controlled, however, growth often is slowed. These children have been found to produce normal to increased amounts of growth hormone, but levels of IGF-I are decreased. The best treatment is to get the diabetes under adequate control.

Growth Hormone Deficiency

This condition is an important cause of short stature but a complicated one. We have devoted chapter 10 to describing the characteristics, causes, and diagnosis of growth hormone deficiency.

UNDERNUTRITION

Some children are short simply because they are not eating an adequate quantity or variety of foods. The causes and consequences of undernutrition are discussed in chapter 3.

CDC Growth Charts: United States

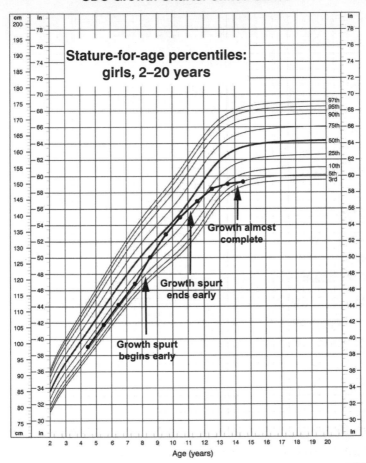

Stature-for-age percentiles: girls, 2–20 years

Age (years)

Modified from NCHS growth charts:
Published May 30, 2000.
SOURCE: Developed by the National Center for Health Statistics in collaboration with
the National Center for Chronic Disease Prevention and Health Promotion (2000).

Figure 9. Growth chart of a girl with early puberty. This girl grew along the 10th percentile during childhood. She then experienced early puberty, causing an early growth spurt starting at about eight years old. As a result, her height climbed almost to the 50th percentile. However, her growth also stopped sooner than most girls; so by age 14, her growth is essentially complete at an adult height close to the 5th percentile.

95

CHRONIC DISEASE

As discussed previously, a large number of chronic diseases can impact a child's growth. Often, the diagnosis of the underlying disease is either made or suspected by the primary care physician, and the child is referred to the appropriate specialist. We cannot discuss all these diseases, but we will briefly explore some of the more important ones that can affect growth with relatively few symptoms to initially suggest the correct diagnosis.

Gastrointestinal Diseases

• **Inflammatory bowel disease** (including Crohn's disease and ulcerative colitis) often impairs growth. Inflammatory bowel disease often causes crampy abdominal pain, diarrhea, decreased appetite, poor weight gain, blood-tinged or dark-colored bowel movements, and/or iron deficiency anemia. However, some children with inflammatory bowel disease will show decreased growth in weight and/or height but few or no gastrointestinal symptoms. If the diagnosis of inflammatory bowel disease is suspected, the primary care doctor will usually refer the child to a pediatric GI specialist.

• **Celiac disease** can also cause growth problems out of proportion to bowel symptoms. This condition is due to a reaction of the intestines to gluten, a protein found in grains such as wheat, barley, and rye. The lining of the intestines becomes injured, which decreases food absorption. Often, these children develop foul-smelling, loose stools and a swollen abdomen. In recent years, a number of studies have reported that 2 to 8 percent of short children *without any GI symptoms* have celiac disease. For this reason, many growth specialists have started ordering blood tests for celiac disease in all children who have significant, unexplained short stature. If the test is positive, the child is usually referred to a pediatric GI specialist who, after confirming the diagnosis, will place the child on a gluten-free diet. This usually causes a significant improvement in growth.

Kidney Disorders

- **Chronic renal failure.** Short stature can be a significant problem for children with this problem. When the kidneys are not functioning properly, chemicals that are normally excreted by the kidneys build up in the blood, causing medical problems, including poor growth. However, it is uncommon for renal failure to be suspected based simply on a child's growth pattern. Most children will have other clues—such as decreased production of urine, blood or protein in the urine, or elevated blood pressure—that will lead to the diagnosis. They are then usually referred to a pediatric nephrologist (kidney specialist). These children often grow significantly faster when given growth hormone, as discussed further in chapter 11.

- **Renal tubular acidosis** can also result in poor growth. This is a condition in which the kidney is unable to hold on to a chemical in the blood called bicarbonate. Excessive loss of bicarbonate in the urine leads to higher-than-normal acid levels in the blood, which can slow growth in height and weight. This problem is something children are usually born with and is generally discovered in the first two years of life. Treatment with medication to replace the lost bicarbonate can help these children grow more normally.

Other Chronic Diseases

Poor growth can occur with many other chronic diseases, including cystic fibrosis, liver disease, severe anemia, HIV infection, and congenital heart disease, to name just a few. Children with these disorders should generally be treated by appropriate pediatric subspecialists.

MEDICATIONS

Some of the medications used to treat chronic health problems in children can affect growth. Two categories in particular are frequently associated with poor growth in height: corticosteroids and stimulant medications.

Corticosteroids

As discussed in chapter 4, a corticosteroid is a type of steroid medication that acts like cortisol, a hormone from the adrenal glands. Many synthetic corticosteroids are used to treat disease: hydrocortisone, cortisone, prednisone, methylprednisolone, and dexamethasone, to name just a few. To make matters even more confusing, each of these medications has both a generic name and one or more brand names. Various corticosteroids can be administered in many ways, including via pill, oral liquid, injection, inhaler, nose spray, or skin cream. If your child is on a medication and you are not sure whether it is a corticosteroid, ask your physician.

If the drug is given for a short time—say, a few days to a week, perhaps to treat an asthma flare-up—there is minimal effect on growth. Sometimes, however, corticosteroids are used repeatedly or continuously for months and even years in children with severe asthma, Crohn's disease, chronic joint disease (arthritis), kidney disease, and other disorders. Corticosteroids, if used repeatedly or for extended periods of time, can slow growth in height. The child's weight, in contrast, will often increase. In addition, corticosteroids can cause other signs and symptoms of Cushing syndrome (see chapter 4). The likelihood that a child receiving corticosteroid treatment will develop growth problems depends on a number of factors, including:

- **The exact medication.** Some are more powerful than others.
- **The dose.** Higher doses carry a greater risk.
- **The route.** Pills, oral liquids, and injections carry a greater risk, but slowing of growth can sometimes occur with other routes such as inhalers (often for asthma), skin creams, and nasal sprays.
- **Duration.** A single short course (a few days) of pills is unlikely to cause growth problems, but children who

receive corticosteroids for many months or years, or whose medical problem requires them to take frequent short courses of these medications, are more likely to have growth problems.

Most physicians treating such children do their best to keep the dose of the corticosteroid as low as possible while still controlling the underlying disease, but when the condition flares up, increases in dose are often necessary. If the inflammation can be controlled by giving corticosteroids on an every-other-day schedule, there may be less effect on growth.

Corticosteroids can also be delivered to the lungs via inhaler. Inhaled steroids have largely replaced oral corticosteroids in the long-term management of asthma. Because inhaled corticosteroids are delivered directly to the lungs, there are fewer effects on the rest of the body. However, a number of carefully done studies have found that inhaled corticosteroids can affect growth, though usually not to the extent of high doses of oral prednisone. It also appears that the effect in many children is temporary. In children with moderate and severe asthma, the very real risk of the disease often outweighs the risk of growth problems or other side effects.

If you are worried that corticosteroids may be interfering with your child's growth, do *not* just discontinue the medication on your own. Stopping the medication can cause the treated disease to flare up and can also cause a serious problem called adrenal insufficiency. Instead, discuss the risks and benefits of the medication with your child's physician. If you still have concerns, consider getting a second opinion, especially from a pediatric specialist who has expertise in your child's disorder.

Stimulant Medications

Attention deficit disorder and attention deficit with hyperactivity disorder are often treated with stimulants; these medications tend, in general, to speed up physical and mental processes. In children with ADD and ADHD, they often increase the attention span and improve school performance. This group of drugs includes many medications, which are usually referred to by their brand names, including Ritalin, Concerta, Dexedrine, Metadate, and Adderall. There is evidence that stimulants used to treat ADD may decrease growth in weight and height. A recent study found that there was on average a 2-centimeter smaller gain in height (20 percent reduction) during the first 24 months in a group of children treated medically for ADHD compared with a nonmedicated control group, as well as a reduction in weight gain. Over the last 10 years, one of the authors has evaluated about 50 children whose growth charts showed slowing of growth in height at or around the time of starting one of these medications. On the other hand, a large number of children take these medications without any obvious effect on growth, so there may be a subset of children who are more susceptible to growth suppression. Because these medications commonly reduce appetite, it is often thought that their effect on height is due to the decrease in weight gain. However, this is not certain, because some children on ADD medications who experience slowing of linear growth are not underweight for their height. Thus there may be other, poorly understood reasons for the effect of these medications on height gain. Although short-term studies have found a variable but definite slowing of growth in the initial phases of treatment with stimulant medications, there are not enough good long-term studies to know whether these medications affect the child's eventual adult height.

If your child is taking a stimulant for ADD and has experienced decreased growth in height or weight, you should discuss this issue with your child's physician. Sometimes a change can be made in the specific medication chosen, the dose, or the timing of doses. Some children may do well without the medications on weekends and during vacations; this may reduce the growth-slowing effects. Some children may do well if switched to Strattera, a newer nonstimulant drug used for ADD. In our opinion, however, there are cases when some slowing of growth must be tolerated because the medication is having a beneficial effect on the child's ability to focus and learn in school and because lower doses and other medications will not suffice. The benefits of a drug must be carefully balanced against the risks. If you are faced with these difficult decisions, discuss them with your child's physician, and if you are still concerned, you may wish to get a second opinion from a child psychiatrist or other specialist in these disorders.

IDIOPATHIC SHORT STATURE

Sometimes we see children in clinic with significant short stature, but we are unable to identify a specific cause despite a careful medical evaluation, including laboratory tests. We refer to this condition as idiopathic short stature. *Idiopathic* is just a fancy word to indicate that we do not understand the cause. Sometimes the child and another family member are both unusually short. In this case, we suspect a genetic cause, but we sometimes cannot identify the specific gene or genes responsible. Gradually, over the years, more and more causes of decreased growth are discovered. However, there is still much that we do not understand about short stature, and many children coming to see the pediatric endocrinologist will fall into the category of idiopathic short stature.

KEY POINTS TO KEEP IN MIND

Most short children are healthy. They are usually short either because they are maturing more slowly than most children or because they come from short families. Less often, however, short stature can be caused by an important medical problem. Many different kinds of illness can impair growth. Sometimes the underlying medical problem is obvious, but other times children have poor growth because of a subtle, unrecognized medical problem.

CHAPTER 8

The Physical, Social, and Psychological Impact of Short Stature

IS SHORT STATURE A PROBLEM?

In previous chapters, we discussed the fact that while some children are short because of an underlying medical problem, more often there is no underlying illness. Most short kids and short adults are healthy. Consequently, when we evaluate short children in our clinic, we can often give the family good news—*Your child is healthy.* For some families, that is all they want to know.

However, for many families, particularly when the child is unusually short, the next question is: *What can we do to treat the short stature?* These parents come to us with the belief that short stature per se is a problem. They believe that being short is stressful to the child, and that any treatment that has a chance of improving the child's growth will have significant psychological benefit and will be worth the effort and expense. Some parents tell us that they seek our help because they fear that their short children will blame them when they end up as short adults, and will wonder why their parents didn't seek treatment for them when they were young enough to benefit.

Are these beliefs valid? Do short people have important problems in life, either in childhood or in adulthood? Do they encounter physical problems, such as difficulty driving a car? Do they face discrimination in their careers or social life? Does short stature cause psychological problems? Does it affect quality of life?

These questions are very controversial and difficult to answer with certainty, but they are important. If we are considering treating short stature, we need to know what exactly we are trying to do. We should know whether there is a problem, and, if so, whether treatment will help it. These issues lie at the core of the debate over the use of growth hormone in short children.

In this chapter, we will first discuss the physical problems that short people in our society encounter, and how short you have to be to experience them. We will address the issue of whether any prejudice against short people exists in terms of finding jobs or mates. We will then explore the controversial question of whether being short by itself causes psychological problems for children, and how parents can help their child successfully adapt to being short. We will emphasize that one of the most important issues is not the child's actual size relative to peers but how the child has adjusted to his or her size.

PHYSICAL CONSEQUENCES OF SHORT STATURE

A very short woman, particularly one who is well under 5 feet tall, may experience some challenges living in a world designed for taller people. She may have to stand on a stool to reach shelves or even to operate a fax machine. She may also be at a disadvantage competing in certain sports. Shopping for clothes may require more effort. The shortest women may need some adaptive equipment to drive a car.

A man of 5 feet, 3 inches, is shorter than 99 percent of adult males. As a result, he may have some of the same challenges that face a very short woman. It may take extra effort to find clothes that fit. He may be at a disadvantage competing in certain sports. However, at 5 feet, 3 inches, he is not far below the average height of women, and so he should not have more difficulty than most women of normal height in driving a car, reaching items on low shelves, or seeing where he's going in a crowd.

Occasionally, someone may be interested in a particular job that requires a minimum physical size, such as being a policeman. For some jobs, this may be an unfair restriction that should be contested. For a very few jobs, physical size may indeed be a factor to consider. However, this consideration is not unique to stature; there are many jobs and careers in the world, and we must pick our path taking into account all of our attributes, including our size, strength, intelligence, specific talents, and preferences.

For children, the physical consequence that seems to cause the most concern is related to sports. Short children are at some disadvantage playing certain sports, such as basketball. Still, there are also many sports in which height is not a major issue, and even in basketball some shorter individuals can excel, usually playing as guards.

Thus, the physical consequences of short stature primarily affect only very short individuals, and even then, most people adjust well. These issues may cause inconvenience and annoyance, but they are generally not insurmountable obstacles in life.

SOCIAL CONSEQUENCES IN ADULTHOOD

We humans have a tendency to judge each other unfairly. We are particularly harsh if another person looks different from us. There is prejudice based on race, gender, religion, and ethnicity. There is also prejudice against people who are obese, have unusual facial appearances, and in some cases against people who are short. Psychological studies designed to isolate these tendencies have shown evidence that people tend to associate taller stature with greater social status and success. As a result, for some people, first impressions may be biased by height. Fortunately, first impressions are usually followed by second and third impressions when additional information about the person becomes available. So the tall man may make a more favorable impression when he walks in the room, but if he opens his mouth and reveals that he is a bore, his height advantage may amount to very little.

Some studies have suggested that income may be related to height. For example, one study reported that men and women in the lowest 10th percentile of the height distribution earned 4 to 5 percent less than those who were between the 20th and 80th percentiles. However, not all studies have shown this effect, particularly when age and education are taken into account. In any case, any possible effect of height on income appears to be weaker than the effects of other factors such as an individual's level of education.

Short men often feel that their ability to date and marry women, particularly taller women, is affected by their stature. However, studies have not found a consistent relationship between height of adult males and their *overall* probability of being married.

The tendency to prejudge people based on their height, sometimes called heightism, is deplorable. It is, in our opinion, similar to racism and sexism, and we should try vigilantly to identify it in ourselves and our society and to eradicate it. If we could do this, far fewer families would come to the doctor asking for treatment for short stature. Our society has begun to recognize and address prejudice related to race, ethnicity, religion, and physical disabilities. We must also recognize and address prejudice against people who are short, tall, or overweight, or have unusual facial appearances or other physical differences.

SOCIAL CONSEQUENCES IN CHILDHOOD

Short children may appear to be younger than their actual age, and as a result others may treat them as they would a younger child. This tendency is referred to as juvenilization. Very short children are sometimes subjected to teasing about their height from their peers. There is evidence that short children experience more bullying than do taller children. Smaller children may be more likely to suffer physical or verbal aggression from their peers, and this can lead to overprotectiveness on the part of parents and teachers. It has been suggested that, in some children, juvenilization, teasing, and bullying can lead to withdrawal from peers and a preference to spend time with younger children or, in other children, to aggressive behavioral problems to try to compensate for this unfair treatment. But is this really true—and if so, how often does it occur?

A recent study tried to evaluate the social consequences of short stature in childhood. The study systematically examined the popularity, friendships, and reputation among peers of a large sample of 6th through 12th graders. Children in the study spanned the range from short to normal to tall, and each child was rated on a number of measures by a group of classroom peers. The authors reported that the child's height was not related to his or her popularity or the number of friendships that the child had. The only measure in which the shorter children were different was that they were rated by their peers as "looking younger" than their normal-size classmates. This study, which differed from many others in looking at short children drawn from the community, suggests that most short children do not suffer serious social problems based on their height. Many previous studies may have found different results because they only looked at children who came to a clinic for evaluation of short stature, an issue that we will discuss later.

PSYCHOLOGICAL CONSEQUENCES IN CHILDHOOD

Some but not all studies have found psychological problems associated with short stature, but the differences between short and normal-size children have not been impressive. For example, one study involved 180 boys and 78 girls undergoing a growth evaluation. The children and their parents were asked a battery of questions about behavioral problems and perceptions of their social adjustment. The short girls had results virtually identical to those of a comparison group of children with normal height in terms of their social competency and behavioral issues. Short boys were described by parents as having somewhat less social competence and more emotional problems than normal-size boys; the boys described themselves as less socially active, but with no more behavioral problems than boys of normal height. Another study, involving 41 short children, also reported that there were no evident, important psychological problems.

As mentioned previously, we must keep in mind that

psychological studies of short children have been done in two different ways. Studies that include only short children who were referred to specialists for evaluation and possible treatment of short stature are examining a select group of children. These children are more likely to be unhappy about their size, and some of the families probably came to the clinic because they wanted something done about their child's growth. It is not clear, however, that findings from this type of study can be generalized to the larger group of short children who are not seen by growth specialists.

The Wessex Growth Study, done in Great Britain, examined short (below the 3rd percentile) healthy children drawn from the community, not the clinic, excluding those with a known disease. Each child was compared with a classmate of normal height. Although some minor psychological differences were noted, these researchers found no evidence of serious psychological problems or academic difficulties in the short children. For example, the self-esteem of the short children was equivalent to that seen in children of normal height. They did find that short children were generally less happy with their height. In other words, the short children wanted to be taller, but the dissatisfaction about height did not have significant effects on other areas of their emotional well-being. This study is quite reassuring. However, one significant limitation is that most of the children studied were between the 1st and 3rd percentiles. Thus, the study tells us about children with mild short stature, but its conclusions may not apply to those with more severe short stature.

We have seen in our own clinical experience numerous short children who, while aware of their shortness relative to their peers, seem well adjusted, maintain many friendships, and participate fully in various age-appropriate activities including sports. Attending school with the same group of peers over many years seems to help, as does having a close and supportive family environment. Perhaps these children are born with a more positive outlook on life in general. These children often ignore any teasing, or at least they do not let it get to them. Although many wish they were taller, they usually don't feel sorry for themselves. For such well-adjusted short children who have no medical explanation for their stature, a heavy parental and physician focus on the child's height and the need to treat it may in some cases be counterproductive—it suggests to children that they are different from others, not "normal."

On the other hand, we have also seen many children in our clinic who tell us that they are distressed about their short stature. Boys are often more distressed than girls, perhaps because people tend to view large size and strength as masculine qualities. Why do we keep seeing children who are distressed by their stature when several research studies suggest that shortness does not cause significant psychological problems? We can imagine several possibilities. First, some of these children are shorter than those in the studies. However, this cannot be the only explanation, because some of the distressed children we see are only mildly short and because some studies suggest that the degree of distress in the child is not related to degree of shortness. A second possibility is that some children may be unusually sensitive psychologically to their physical difference. Third, some children may be quite unhappy about their short stature yet functioning well as a whole; thus they would test well in a psychological study. Finally, some children may be unhappy about other life circumstances such as family, peer-related, or academic problems, but they tend to focus on their short stature as a major cause of their unhappiness to the exclusion of other factors.

WHAT CAN PARENTS DO TO HELP THEIR SHORT CHILD COPE BETTER?

• **Be sensitive to your child's situation but not overprotective.** We suggest that you convey a positive outlook. Be careful not to give your child the idea that short stature is a major disability or something to be ashamed of. If your child believes that short stature is a major handicap, it may well end up being true. Try to teach optimism and self-confidence.

• **Help your child find positive experiences from which to draw strength.** Help him or her discover and cultivate talents, whether in academics, music, art, athletics, or other areas. If he or she is discouraged because of difficulties participating in sports in which size is a major factor, encourage sports such as gymnastics, wrestling, soccer, and swimming. Help your child recognize his or her strengths and fine qualities, perhaps persistence or the ability to understand other people's feelings.

• **Help your child find a supportive peer group.** Sometimes this can be found in the school or neighborhood. Other times, it may be a community group such as the Cub Scouts, a karate class at the YMCA, or a summer camp. These groups can help build feelings of self-esteem and acceptance.

• **Be alert for signs of behavioral problems.** Some short children may cope with their size difference by manifesting more immature or clowning behavior so that their behavior is size-appropriate rather than age-appropriate. Others tend to be adopted by a group of larger children, often to protect against bullying, and end up becoming the group mascot. Still others may respond with aggressive behavior. You can discuss better coping strategies with your child. For example, you may want to point out that getting angry when teased about size tends to encourage other children to persist in the teasing, and that learning to ignore it or to simply walk away is a better strategy.

• **Consider consulting a child psychologist or psychiatrist.** This is especially important if your child is distressed by teasing or juvenilization, or is otherwise having psychological problems. If a child can learn to cope more effectively with teasing and other height-related problems through counseling, he or she may see an improvement in the quality of life greater than any benefit from growth hormone treatment. We must admit that, to our knowledge, no rigorous studies have been done to see how effective psychological intervention is in these situations. However, we think that if your child is having significant problems adapting to being short, you should consider counseling, whether or not you are also considering medical treatment.

KEY POINTS TO KEEP IN MIND

Overall, we think that the data from psychological studies are reassuring. Short stature may be unpleasant for children, who may sometimes be bullied or otherwise treated unfairly. However, the studies suggest that most children with short stature do not experience serious social isolation or serious psychological problems. These findings may help some parents relax a bit. In contrast, some studies focusing on children *referred for* evaluation of short stature, rather than taken from the general population, do report some increased problems with emotional adjustment and behavior, especially in boys. Overall, however, the studies suggest that for most children, the consequences of short stature may not be as bad as parents may fear. Yet for some children—particularly those who are either very short or not coping well with other aspects of their lives—there may be reason for concern.

CHAPTER 9

How Specialists Evaluate Short Children

In chapter 7, we learned that short stature can be caused by many different disorders. How, then, does a growth specialist sort through this long list to determine the cause in an individual child? It's much like detective work. We ask a lot of questions, we examine the physical evidence, and we rely on the lab for technical help. When clues emerge, we follow up on each lead. In this chapter, we'll discuss this process to help you know what to expect if you and your child's physician decide that your child needs to be evaluated by a specialist. We'll also give you some suggestions about how to make the visit to the specialist productive.

SELECTING AN APPROPRIATE DOCTOR

If the level of concern about a short child is low, many primary care physicians (family practitioners and pediatricians) will handle the situation themselves. Sometimes, they will increase the frequency of height and weight checks or order a limited number of tests. However, as the level of concern increases, primary care physicians will often refer the patient for further evaluation. Even pediatricians—specialists in child health—will refer kids to a subspecialist if the growth pattern appears abnormal and the cause has not been determined.

Which type of specialist is most appropriate? Often the choice will depend on the specific situation. For example, if a child has poor growth, abdominal pain, and intermittent diarrhea, a referral to a pediatric gastroenterologist (subspecialist for stomach and intestinal problems, also known as a GI specialist) would be appropriate. If the child has poor growth and some birth defects or an unusual appearance, the primary care provider may refer to a geneticist. Similarly, depending on the clinical situation, a child may be referred to a pediatric cardiologist (subspecialist for heart problems), a pediatric pulmonologist (subspecialist for lung problems), a pediatric nephrologist (subspecialist for kidney problems), a pediatric rheumatologist (subspecialist for joint problems), a pediatric neurologist (subspecialist for brain problems), a child psychiatrist (if anorexia nervosa is suspected), or another subspecialist.

If, as is frequently the case, there are no clinical clues pointing in a specific direction, and the primary care physician is concerned, the child is usually referred to a pediatric endocrinologist. Pediatric endocrinologists specialize in diseases that involve hormones. In general, they have completed three years of general pediatrics training and an additional three years of fellowship training in pediatric endocrinology at an academic medical center, where they worked under the supervision of several senior people in the field. Other than childhood diabetes, growth problems are the most common conditions referred to the pediatric endocrinologist, so they will have acquired much experience in this area.

FINDING A PEDIATRIC ENDOCRINOLOGIST

How should a family locate a pediatric endocrinologist? In most large cities, there are several of them at major medical centers, often associated with a university. Most of the primary care physicians in the area have referred previous patients to these centers, and will often have one center and perhaps specific pediatric endocrinologists that they prefer. Some larger cities also have one or more pediatric endocrinologists in private practice. Problems finding a pediatric endocrinologist most often occur when the family lives in a town or small city that is far from the nearest academic medical center and too small to support a pediatric endocrinologist. In such situations, it may be tempting to see an adult endocrinologist rather than travel long distances to a city with a pediatric endocrinology specialist. However, adult endocrinologists (who generally refer to themselves simply as endocrinologists) are trained in internal medicine, rather than pediatrics, followed by subspecialty training that focuses primarily on endocrine disease in adulthood. While there are some adult endocrinologists who do a good job evaluating short children, most have much less training in growth disorders, and we feel that consulting a pediatric endocrinologist is usually worth any extra travel.

How can you tell if the pediatric endocrinologist closest to you or the one to whom you have been referred is well trained? Hopefully, your child's primary care physician will know the local pediatric endocrinologists and will have chosen one that he or she trusts. It is also reassuring if the pediatric endocrinologist is board-certified in pediatric endocrinology, indicating the successful completion of training in pediatric endocrinology and of a certifying exam. Board certification does not guarantee that the pediatric endocrinologist is a good clinician, but it's a good sign. Conversely, some skilled pediatric endocrinologists are not board-certified for various reasons.

To determine whether a particular physician is board-certified in pediatric endocrinology or to search for a board-certified pediatric endocrinologist near you, go to the Web site of the American Board of Pediatrics, www.abp.org.

WHY DOES IT TAKE SO LONG TO GET AN APPOINTMENT?

Once parents have decided to take their child to a pediatric endocrinologist, they are often dismayed to learn that there are no appointments available for three or more months. Unfortunately, there are not enough pediatric endocrinologists in many parts of the country to accommodate the high demand for consultations.

Although it is frustrating to have to wait so long for an evaluation, in the large majority of cases doing so will not significantly impact the child's health. You may be worried that a delay in treatment will decrease your child's eventual adult height. In most cases, waiting a few months will have a negligible effect on adult height. However, there may be a need for haste if you suspect that your child is growing poorly because of a serious underlying disease. If you think that there might be some reason for urgency in your child's case, talk to your primary care physician, who either will reassure you or, if he or she agrees, may call the endocrinologist to explain the reason for the urgency.

Usually, seeing a skilled specialist in whom you have confidence is more important than seeing someone quickly. However, you do want to be sure that when your appointment finally arrives, you have done everything you can to make the visit as productive as possible. That is the focus of the next section.

MAKING THE MOST OF YOUR VISIT TO A GROWTH SPECIALIST

Collecting Growth Information

Sometimes, when we are seeing a child in our clinic for short stature and we ask the parents for the copy of the child's growth chart, we are met by a puzzled look. "No one told us that we needed to bring it," they tell us, or "Our doctor said he faxed it to your office" (which often means three or more months ago). By this point, you probably understand that a key part of any growth evaluation is a review of the growth chart. It shows us how the child ended up where he or she is now. We strongly suggest that you obtain a copy of your child's growth chart from your regular pediatrician and carry it with you to the appointment, rather than hope that it will be mailed or faxed in a timely fashion and actually end up in the hands of the specialist at the time of your visit. Also remember that some of us practice out of more than one office; the growth chart we need could be sitting in an office 20 miles away from where we are seeing your child. In some cases, the physician who refers a short child has seen him or her on only one occasion, while the bulk of the growth records are in the file of the previous pediatrician who may be in another city. In that case, the parents should contact this previous pediatrician and request that the growth chart and any possibly useful lab tests be mailed to the *parents*—not to the specialist. Because this process may take weeks, make the request well before the time of the growth consultation. We should also mention that most children older than age 3 should have two growth charts, one spanning birth to 3 years, and the other covering the interval from 2 to 18 years. If your child is young, try to obtain both growth charts. If your child is older—say, 10 years old—the chart showing growth before age 3 is less critical but still may be helpful if it's available.

Two other sources of growth information should not be ignored, especially if the child has not had regular well-child visits. Some school systems have nurses measure and weigh children once or twice a year, and these records can help fill in the gaps. Also, some parents have records of home measurements made on a wall or door. While perhaps not as accurate as those obtained with a stadiometer in a doctor's office (see chapter 5), home measurements can provide additional useful information when records from the pediatrician are scant.

What Family History Should Be Collected?

As discussed earlier, most children who are short have either genetic short stature or constitutional growth delay, and a good family history can provide important clues to these diagnoses. Be ready to provide the pediatric endocrinologist with the heights of the child's parents (biological, not adoptive or stepparents), the grandparents, and older, fully grown siblings. For brothers and sisters who are still growing, height percentiles should be obtained if possible. Note should be made of any aunts, uncles, cousins, and great-grandparents who are or were unusually short. In addition, the timing of puberty for close relatives is important. For older girls and women, the age at menarche (the time of the first menstrual period) is a good indicator of whether puberty was delayed. The average is about 12 to 13 years, so menarche after age 14 indicates that puberty was delayed. For boys and men, there is no one event that defines the timing of puberty. However, some fathers will recall the year during which they had a growth spurt and shot up 4 inches or more. In the average boy, this occurs between 13 and 14, so a growth spurt after age 15 can be considered delayed. Since most boys are done growing by 16 or 17, any father who recalls that he grew even an inch after graduating from high school probably had delayed puberty. Some fathers simply recall that they matured somewhat later than their peers without being able to put a precise age on it. Other parents will recall that they were short as children but then, during their teen years, caught up with and surpassed many of their peers, and this information is also useful.

Parents should also bring to the visit information concerning close relatives who have any important medical conditions. Some disorders run in families, so if a close relative has hypothyroidism, for example, this information will raise the endocrinologist's level of suspicion that your child might have the same problem.

Previous Laboratory Tests, X-Rays, and Medical Evaluations

Some children will not have received any laboratory tests or X-rays in the past. However, if your child has had lab work or a bone age done as part of an evaluation for stature, try to bring these results with you. Many pediatric endocrinologists want to interpret the bone age themselves. If a child has been evaluated by another pediatric endocrinologist or by another physician for any problems that might be related to growth, you should try to bring the records with you, including the physician's notes or dictated letters.

Should the Primary Care Physician Order Tests Before a Specialist Visit?

If the primary care physician suspects that a growth problem might be caused by a particular disorder, then he or she may order tests related to that specific problem. The result might determine which subspecialist the primary care physician refers the child to. However, if the primary care physician does not suspect a particular disorder and has decided to refer the child to a pediatric endocrinologist, ordering tests, in our experience, is usually not helpful. In addition, if the pediatric endocrinologist wants more labs, the child will then have had to endure two needle sticks rather than one. Sometimes, however, the primary care doctor is worried enough to take the time to call the specialist, and the specialist mentions over the phone which tests should be done before the visit. Often, getting a hand X-ray for a bone age is helpful. Because many pediatric endocrinologists like to read these X-rays themselves rather than rely on the reading of the radiologist, bring with you a copy of the actual X-ray—not just the written report.

Table 7. What To Bring to the Pediatric Endocrinologist's Office

Growth charts—as complete as possible
Family information:
    Heights
    Timing of puberty
    Medical problems
Previous results:
    Laboratory tests
    Bone age X-ray—bring the film
    Physician's notes and letters if relevant to growth

Preparing Your Child for Your Visit to a Growth Specialist

It is not unusual for children to be anxious about visiting a new physician, particularly if they are very sensitive about the fact that they are short. They may be worried that a serious medical problem will be uncovered. It is helpful if the child can be provided with some simple information as to the purpose of the visit and what it will entail. You can point out that most short children are healthy and will do fine if they are left alone and given time to grow. However, the purpose of your visit is to make sure there is not an underlying problem that might require further testing and respond to treatment. The specific possibility of growth hormone treatment should not be played up; the majority of short children we see are not really in need of growth hormone and would benefit little if it were given.

If you are seeing a specialist at a university medical center, you and your child should be aware that you may encounter people in various stages of their training, from medical students to pediatric residents to fellows training in pediatric endocrinology. Sometimes these trainees work alongside the doctor. Sometimes they will be the first person to talk to you and your child, and they will then bring in the specialist to review what they have learned. The specialist will then explain what he or she thinks should be done and answer any questions you may have.

The child can be told that much of the visit will be spent talking about the medical history and reviewing any information brought from the office of the referring doctor. Many doctors will want to know how the child feels about his or her size and how much teasing or being pushed around he or she experiences. If the child has been sensitive in the past about undressing and having a complete exam, you may want to discuss these concerns and try to allay any embarrassment.

THE DAY OF THE VISIT

The pediatric endocrinologist will usually ask about your child's birth, current and prior illnesses, and medications. He or she will want to review the growth chart that you brought to understand the child's pattern of growth. The endocrinologist will probably ask about the height, timing of puberty, and illnesses in other family members. He or she may ask certain specific questions to be sure nothing is missed: "Does your child have abdominal pain or diarrhea?" "How is the nutritional intake?" In addition, the doctor will probably want to know how your child feels about his or her height.

Next comes the physical exam. Often a nurse will have already obtained the height using a stadiometer, as well as recording weight, pulse, and blood pressure. Many doctors will remeasure the height themselves to be certain it's accurate. The doctor will then do a physical exam, looking for any clues to the cause of the short stature, though in the majority of cases the exam will be normal.

LABORATORY TESTS TO EVALUATE SHORT STATURE

There is a great deal of variability as to how many tests different pediatric endocrinologists will order after seeing a short child, so your experience may be different from the approach we generally take. Some specialists order the same list of tests on nearly all short children they see; others often order no tests at all if a child seems healthy and has been growing at a normal rate. Experienced specialists can often make a diagnosis of genetic short stature and constitutional growth delay without any blood tests, based on the history, growth chart, and the normal physical exam. In many situations, however, judicious ordering of tests can make an important diagnosis or at least help exclude several possibilities.

When Is Laboratory Testing Needed?

Some children are only slightly short, healthy, have similarly short parents, and are growing parallel to the normal percentile curves. In these situations, we can generally reassure the parents that the likelihood of a significant underlying disease is very low. We do not usually need to do many or perhaps any tests. Sometimes we will just order a bone age to help identify constitutional delay of growth and predict height. Other times, we see children who are unusually short or who have a worrisome pattern on the growth chart. For some of these children, we already have a good explanation: Perhaps there is an illness, a medication, or a family background sufficient to explain the growth pattern. However, sometimes the child's degree of short stature or growth pattern is worrisome, but after the medical history and physical exam, we do not have an explanation. We will refer to this situation as "important, unexplained short stature." This is the child who most needs a broad laboratory evaluation. Some of the common tests are listed in table 8.

Table 8. Screening Tests That May Be Ordered

Routine blood chemistry tests
Blood count
Erythrocyte sedimentation rate
Thyroid tests
Insulin-like growth factor I and IGF-binding protein 3
Tests for celiac disease
Urinalysis
Karyotype (chromosome analysis)
Bone age X-ray

Routine Blood Chemistry Tests

One set of blood tests often performed to evaluate short stature is called a Comprehensive Metabolic Panel (although it has different names at different medical centers). This is a bundle of about 14 to 20 common tests run as a group. Included are tests for common chemicals in the blood such as sodium, potassium, chloride, and bicarbonate; measures of kidney function (blood urea nitrogen, or BUN, as well as creatinine); measures of bone health (calcium and an enzyme from bone called alkaline phosphatase); and measures of liver health (the blood protein called albumin—which is made in the liver—and certain enzymes that can leak out of a damaged liver).

Blood Count

Another lab test that is commonly ordered is the complete blood count (CBC). Anemia (low red blood cell count) severe enough to cause poor growth without other symptoms is rare, but the finding of milder anemia could be a clue to an underlying problem, such as inflammatory bowel disease or celiac disease. As mentioned in chapters 3 and 7, these diseases can cause falloff in growth without many symptoms related to the bowels. The anemia can be due to iron deficiency if patients are either losing blood in their stools or not absorbing iron from the food in their intestines.

Erythrocyte Sedimentation Rate (ESR)

The ESR—a measure of how fast red blood cells settle to the bottom of a blood sample—is an imperfect but useful indicator of inflammation in the body. An elevated ESR can sometimes be a useful clue in detecting inflammatory bowel disease and other inflammatory conditions.

Thyroid Tests

Only a small number of children are short because they are not making enough thyroid hormone. However, because this condition is usually quite easy to diagnose or exclude with simple blood tests, and because it is readily treatable, thyroid tests are ordered in nearly every short child who has blood drawn. There are two separate tests, which need to be looked at together. First, the lab will measure the amount of thyroid hormone in the blood, either the total amount of thyroid hormone (variously called thyroxine, T_4, total thyroxine, or total T_4), or a more accurate test called free T_4, which measures only the thyroid hormone that is "free" (not bound to blood proteins). The other important test is called TSH. As discussed in chapter 7, this pituitary hormone typically increases in response to a failing thyroid gland, so that when the thyroid gland is underactive, we see a low total or free T_4 and a high TSH.

If the total or free T_4 comes back low but the TSH is normal (not elevated), this could indicate that the pituitary is not able to make enough TSH to maintain normal thyroid hormone production; when the pituitary is healthy, a low T_4 would normally trigger an increase in TSH. If there is a deficiency of TSH in a short child, chances are increased that a deficiency of growth hormone will eventually be found.

Insulin-like Growth Factor I (IGF-I)

As discussed in chapter 4, IGF-I is the growth factor that mediates many of the effects of growth hormone on growth, and thus its blood levels tend to be lower than normal if the body is not producing a normal amount of growth hormone. Growth hormone itself, in blood drawn at the time of a regular doctor visit, is not useful, because, as mentioned earlier, its levels are low during most of the day with brief elevations, especially at night. However, levels of IGF-I are relatively stable, so it doesn't matter what time the test is taken. Because growth hormone stimulates IGF-I, a low IGF-I level suggests growth hormone deficiency. Still, not all children with low IGF-I have such a deficiency. Low IGF-I is also seen in children with poor nutrition and even sometimes in children with constitutional growth delay or idiopathic short stature. Conversely, not all children with growth hormone deficiency have low IGF-I. So IGF-I can be helpful, but it must be interpreted with caution.

IGF-Binding Protein 3 (IGFBP-3)

This test measures a protein produced in the liver that binds to IGF-I in the blood and protects it, keeping it from being quickly broken down. The reason this test is useful in screening for growth hormone deficiency is that, like IGF-I, IGFBP-3 production is under the influence of growth hormone. Thus, when there isn't much growth hormone being made, levels of IGFBP-3 tend to be low. This test is similar to the IGF-I test in that low levels of IGFBP-3 suggest but do not prove growth hormone deficiency; conversely, some children with GH deficiency do not have low IGFBP-3 levels. Like IGF-I, the IGFBP-3 test is sometimes helpful but must be interpreted with caution.

Tests for Celiac Disease

As discussed in the previous chapter, certain bowel disorders can impact a child's growth but may result in few if any symptoms related to bowel function. Because celiac disease can be missed if we test for it only in children with diarrhea or stomach pain, it has become common to screen for this condition in any child being evaluated for important, unexplained short stature or in a child with short stature plus GI symptoms. Two of the tests for celiac disease, called anti-endomysial IgA antibodies and tissue transglutaminase IgA antibodies, are quite accurate (but not perfect), and are rarely positive in children who do not have celiac disease. The blood tests are only screening tests; if they are positive, the next step is usually referral to a pediatric GI specialist, who may perform a small-bowel biopsy to confirm the diagnosis before recommending a gluten-free diet (the treatment for this disorder).

Urinalysis

Sometimes a urine sample is examined to look for evidence of kidney disease. The finding of protein or blood in the urine, though uncommon, would signal the need for an evaluation by a pediatric kidney specialist.

Karyotype

A karyotype is a test to evaluate the child's chromosomes. Recall that the normal number of chromosomes is 46 (23 pairs), including two X chromosomes in girls and an X plus a Y in boys. A karyotype involves studying the appearance of the patient's chromosomes under the microscope. Usually, the chromosomes are obtained from a blood sample.

If a child is unusually short and has other abnormalities suggesting a genetic problem, he or she will often be referred to a geneticist, and a karyotype will usually be performed. In addition, a karyotype is also useful to detect

Turner syndrome in girls. As discussed in chapter 7, some girls with this syndrome will have short stature and few, if any, other signs. Therefore, a pediatric endocrinologist should order a karyotype in girls with important, unexplained short stature, even if they do not have other signs of Turner syndrome.

The karyotype will only detect genetic problems that involve large amounts of DNA. Genetic disease involving small amounts of DNA—say, one gene—cannot be detected by a karyotype. However, advances in molecular biology are steadily expanding the number of genetic diseases that can be detected using other genetic tests.

Bone Age X-Ray

A bone age X-ray is often ordered as part of the evaluation. This X-ray of the left hand and wrist shows how mature the bones appear. The pediatric endocrinologist or radiologist (X-ray specialist) can compare the child's X-ray with an atlas of normal X-rays from children of different ages. If a child has an X-ray that looks most like that of the average 6-year old, we say that the child has a bone age of 6 years. A bone age that's delayed by a year or more is seen with many endocrine and non-endocrine diseases, so it does not, by itself, establish a specific diagnosis. Some delay is also seen in many children with benign forms of short stature such as constitutional delay of growth. A bone age is also useful for height prediction, as discussed in chapter 6.

KEY POINTS TO KEEP IN MIND

If a child has significant short stature, the primary care physician will often refer to a specialist, often a pediatric endocrinologist. You can make the most of your visit to this specialist by bringing with you a growth chart (as complete as possible), previous doctors' notes, lab results and X-rays, and certain medical information about family members. The pediatric endocrinologist will usually ask many questions about your child's health and do a careful physical exam. Depending on the situation, he or she may then order certain laboratory tests to screen for any subtle, underlying disease causing poor growth.

CHAPTER 10

Growth Hormone Deficiency

We are now ready to focus our attention on the one cause of short stature that parents are often most concerned about: growth hormone deficiency. Making the diagnosis of growth hormone deficiency is more complicated than most people realize.

During the 1970s and early 1980s, the diagnosis of growth hormone deficiency was made only when there was strong evidence that GH levels were low. As we will discuss further in chapter 11, the supply of growth hormone was very limited; there was only enough to treat patients who had what we would call severe or "classic" GH deficiency. Studies from that era put the frequency of growth hormone deficiency between 1 in 4,000 and 1 in 10,000 children, meaning it was fairly uncommon. By that estimate, of the children whose height fell below the 3rd percentile, only about 1 in 200 were thought to have growth hormone deficiency. Pediatric endocrinologists practicing in that era developed a pretty good idea of what a child with classic growth hormone deficiency looked like and what type of growth pattern tended to indicate the diagnosis. Children who were somewhat short but growing at a normal rate were generally not even tested for growth hormone deficiency; their parents were simply told that their child had genetic short stature or constitutional growth delay, and that no treatment was needed.

All that began to change in 1985 with the introduction of biosynthetic GH—growth hormone manufactured in a pharmaceutical plant using genetically engineered bacteria. As the GH supply increased, the number of children diagnosed with "growth hormone deficiency" began to climb sharply. In this chapter, we will first describe the characteristics of children with classic growth hormone deficiency and the different causes of it. We will note that the diagnosis of all but the most severe growth hormone deficiency is difficult, because there is no single reliable test for it. Finally, we will offer our view on why growth hormone deficiency has become such a common diagnosis over the past 20 years and why many children currently labeled as growth hormone deficient may not really have this disorder.

CLEAR-CUT GH DEFICIENCY

So how do experienced growth specialists distinguish the occasional child with classic, clear-cut GH deficiency from the large number of short children they evaluate every week? As we discussed previously, the child's growth chart can provide important clues. Children with GH deficiency are typically of normal size at birth. Sometime in the first one or two years of life, they start to grow at a slower-than-normal rate, and their height percentile decreases. Those with the most severe GH deficiency will already be well below the 5th percentile on the growth chart by one or two years of age, while in milder deficiency, the falloff may be more gradual. If their height is tracked over time, they will usually drop farther and farther below the normal range (see figure 10). The weight chart may also show a gradual decline over time, but often weight is less affected than height. Thus, the child with clear-cut growth hormone deficiency is usually not underweight for height and may even be on the chubby side.

In most cases of severe growth hormone deficiency, the parents are not unusually short, which is helpful in excluding the diagnosis of familial short stature. Because relatively few cases of growth hormone deficiency are familial, we don't usually find siblings or close relatives with GH deficiency. During the physical exam, we look for evidence of increased body fat, particularly fat with a ripply appearance around the abdomen and chest; a high-pitched voice; and an immature facial appearance. GH-deficient boys may have a small penis.

Many children with classic, clear-cut growth hormone

CDC Growth Charts: United States

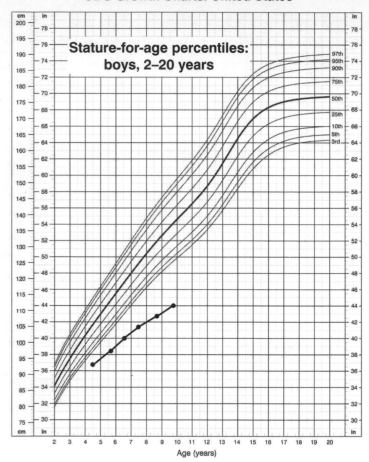

Stature-for-age percentiles:
boys, 2–20 years

Modified from NCHS growth charts:
Published May 30, 2000.
SOURCE: Developed by the National Center for Health Statistics in collaboration with
the National Center for Chronic Disease Prevention and Health Promotion (2000).

Figure 10. Growth chart of a boy with severe, congenital growth hormone deficiency. He was of normal size when born but by age four, he was already well below the normal range. He subsequently continued to fall farther from normal.

deficiency have what we call isolated GH deficiency, meaning there is no evidence of other pituitary hormone deficiencies. Other children have a more general problem with the pituitary gland and are deficient in other pituitary hormones besides GH; such a diagnosis is sometimes suggested when we find that other pituitary hormones are affected.

The most common other pituitary deficiency is thyroid-stimulating hormone (TSH). TSH deficiency causes hypothyroidism, but it is often so mild that it causes few symptoms and can be detected only by blood tests.

Less common is lack of the adrenal-stimulating hormone called ACTH. ACTH deficiency, especially when it is combined with GH deficiency and especially in young children, can cause hypoglycemia (low blood sugar), which, in turn, can cause convulsions (seizures) or periods of unresponsiveness. ACTH deficiency can also cause fatigue, poor appetite, poor weight gain, nausea, or vomiting.

Children with growth hormone deficiency may also be missing two other pituitary hormones called luteinizing hormone (LH) and follicle-stimulating hormone (FSH). These hormones stimulate the gonads—the ovaries or the testes. In a boy, lack of LH may be apparent in infancy because it results in low testosterone production before birth, resulting in an abnormally small penis or undescended testes. In both sexes, LH and FSH are needed for normal puberty, and thus deficiency can cause delayed or absent puberty. However, some problems that cause GH deficiency may cause early puberty.

The final pituitary hormone that may be missing in a child with growth hormone deficiency is called vaso-pressin or antidiuretic hormone. Lack of this hormone causes an inability of the kidneys to conserve water, re-sulting in large amounts of pale urine. The child will usually urinate frequently, may start wetting the bed, and usually needs to drink large amounts frequently to keep up with what is coming out in the urine. This condition is referred to as diabetes insipidus; a pediatrician can do a preliminary test for it by testing an early-morning urine sample. Another initial approach is to have the parents measure the amount of urine the child produces in one day, or measure the amount of liquid that the child drinks in one day. The development of diabetes insipi-dus in a child signals an urgent need for an endocrine evaluation.

CAUSES OF GROWTH HORMONE DEFICIENCY

As mentioned previously, growth hormone deficiency can be classified according to whether it is present from birth (congenital growth hormone deficiency)—the ma-jority of cases—or develops later in childhood (acquired growth hormone deficiency). Many of the principal causes are listed in table 9.

Table 9. Principal Causes of
Growth Hormone Deficiency

Congenital

Idiopathic growth hormone deficiency—no cause identified.

Injury to the hypothalamus or pituitary during birth.

Defects in specific genes responsible for normal pituitary
    development.

Mutations in the gene for growth hormone itself.

Congenital malformations of the brain. The most common is called
    septo-optic dysplasia, which results in visual impairment due to
    small optic nerves and developmental delay.

Acquired

Tumors in the area of the pituitary or the hypothalamus.

Langerhans cell histiocytosis—an infiltration of abnormal cells that
    can cause a rash, bone defects, and/or pituitary problems.

Radiation to the area of the pituitary as part of treatment for a tumor.

Severe head injury.

Causes of Congenital Growth Hormone Deficiency

Although congenital growth hormone deficiency usually has no identifiable cause, sometimes it is associated
with specific birth defects, often involving the brain. In
addition, more and more genes are being identified that
regulate pituitary development and that, if defective, can
result in severe growth hormone deficiency.

Causes of Acquired Growth Hormone Deficiency

The distinction between congenital and acquired
growth hormone deficiency is best made by reviewing the

growth chart. Children with a congenital problem may sometimes grow normally for the first year or so of life but will show a gradual falloff in growth over the next one to three years and are usually extremely short by the time they reach age five to six. The smaller number with acquired growth hormone deficiency usually will have some years of normal growth, followed by a period of slow growth and declining growth percentiles.

Sometimes the cause of acquired growth hormone deficiency is obvious—for example if the child has previously had surgery or radiation treatment in the area of the pituitary gland—but often the cause is not immediately apparent. When we see a growth pattern such as that described above in a short and pudgy child, we always ask about symptoms that might suggest the possibility of a brain tumor, such as headaches that are becoming increasingly frequent and severe. Since the pituitary gland is very close to the optic nerves, loss of vision, especially peripheral vision, is a very worrisome sign. Another worrisome sign is excessive drinking and urination due to diabetes insipidus. It is important to order a brain and pituitary MRI in any child who is diagnosed with growth hormone deficiency that the growth chart suggests is acquired, in order to look for a tumor in the area of the pituitary. We discuss the use of brain imaging again later in this chapter.

The most common tumor causing growth hormone deficiency is called craniopharyngioma, a slowly growing tumor that arises in the area of the pituitary gland. Headaches are common due to the increased pressure inside the skull as the tumor gets larger, and 60 percent of children will have some visual disturbance. A CT scan or MRI is used to detect this and other tumors in the region of the pituitary gland. The usual treatment is surgical removal of as much of the tumor as possible.

Radiation can also cause acquired GH deficiency. Often this occurs in patients who have had tumors in the area of the head and neck that required radiation treatment to an area that included the pituitary gland. Lower doses of radiation typically result in isolated growth hormone deficiency, whereas with higher doses, several pituitary hormones can be affected.

Growth Hormone Insensitivity

This is a rare cause of poor growth. With this condition, the child can make growth hormone, but the child's cells and tissues are unable to respond to it. It is usually due to a mutation in the gene for the GH receptor, the protein needed by cells to respond to the hormone. Children with this condition are typically far below the normal range in height and weight and, when tested, are found to have high levels of growth hormone but low levels of IGF-I. Growth hormone therapy is ineffective, but IGF-I (brand name Increlex) has recently been approved by the Food and Drug Administration for this rare condition.

MAKING THE DIAGNOSIS OF GROWTH HORMONE DEFICIENCY

Unfortunately, there is no simple test that identifies growth hormone deficiency accurately and consistently. Measuring the amount of GH in a single blood sample is not helpful because, as explained earlier, the secretion of growth hormone by the pituitary gland is pulsatile, which means that it can be low for hours, then rise quickly, then drop to a low level again. Measuring the levels of IGF-I and IGFBP-3 (see chapter 9) are better tests, but still not very accurate. Thus they can be used as screening tests to identify children more likely to have growth hormone deficiency, but they cannot by themselves be used to make a definite diagnosis or exclude it. The traditional method for diagnosing growth hormone deficiency has been to use the growth charts, medical history, physical exam, and the IGF-I and possibly IGFBP-3 tests to pick out the children more likely to have GH deficiency as the cause of their slow growth, and then do growth hormone stimulation testing (also known as growth hormone provocative testing) on them.

The theory behind growth hormone stimulation testing is that certain drugs will cause a healthy pituitary gland to release enough growth hormone into the blood to cause GH concentration to rise above a certain level; failure of GH to rise high enough is thus indicative of growth hormone deficiency. In most centers, two such tests are done sequentially, and blood typically is drawn through an IV line approximately every 30 minutes during the tests, with a total of 7 to 10 blood samples drawn over a period of several hours. The medications most commonly used for this test include two of the following: clonidine (a pill usually used to treat high blood pressure), L-dopa (a medication used to treat Parkinson's disease, also given in pill form), arginine (an amino acid given by intravenous infusion), and insulin, which causes a rapid drop in blood sugar and triggers release of growth hormone. These tests are fairly safe, but occasionally we encounter side effects. For example, clonidine often causes mild to moderate drowsiness, and, because it lowers blood pressure, we sometimes see children faint if they stand up too quickly. L-dopa can cause nausea and vomiting. Insulin is the most potentially dangerous of the group, since the fall in blood glucose it produces is sometimes large enough to cause a decline in alertness and occasionally a seizure (convulsion). It requires careful monitoring by the doctor and nurses.

Interpretation of Stimulation Tests

After each stimulation medication is given, the level of growth hormone tends to rise and then decline again. The highest measured value of growth hormone obtained during the test is called the peak growth hormone value. If a child has a peak value over a certain cutoff, we say that the child has passed the test and is not growth hormone deficient. So, for example, if a child's growth hormone increases to 15 ng/ml (levels in blood are measured in units of nanograms per milliliter, abbreviated ng/ml) after taking clonidine and if the doctor uses 10 ng/ml as the cutoff, the doctor would say that the child has passed the test and does not have growth hormone deficiency. What if the peak growth hormone after clonidine was only 5 ng/ml? We would say that the child had "failed" the clonidine test, but most doctors would not yet conclude that GH was deficient. Even normal children often fail to respond to any single stimulation. Therefore, most doctors will not make a diagnosis of growth hormone deficiency unless the child has failed two different stimulation tests (which are usually done one after the other on the same day). So to receive a diagnosis of GH deficiency, all values obtained during both tests must be less than the cutoff value. It all sounds very scientific and precise. Unfortunately, there are many problems with GH testing, which we will enumerate below.

• **What is the cutoff value that defines growth hormone deficiency?** There is no agreed-upon answer, and what doctors tell patients has changed over the years. In the 1960s, the cutoff was 3 ng/ml, which was later raised to 5 and then to 7 ng/ml, where it stayed for many years. In 1985, as biosynthetic growth hormone came on the market, the cutoff was raised at most medical centers to 10 ng/ml. This increase was not based on rigorous scientific evidence. Over the years, several studies have shown that many perfectly healthy children with normal heights and normal rates of growth will fail both growth hormone stimulation tests if a cutoff of 10 or 7 ng/ml is used. This suggests that using a cutoff of 10 (or even 7) labels some short children as having growth hormone deficiency when in fact familial short stature, constitutional growth delay, or some other factor may be causing their shortness. Lowering the cutoff value would decrease the number of children who receive an incorrect diagnosis of growth hormone deficiency. However, it might also increase the number of children who are truly GH deficient but are missed by the tests.

- **Sex steroid priming.** Some specialists in our field believe that sex steroid priming improves the accuracy of growth hormone testing. Typically, a child is given estrogen pills or an injection of testosterone (estrogen and testosterone are both considered sex steroids) before the stimulation tests are done. This sex steroid priming increases growth hormone secretion in the same way that sex steroids increase GH production at the time of puberty. The same short 10-year-old boy or girl who might have a peak growth hormone of 6 ng/ml without sex steroid priming might have a peak growth hormone of 15 ng/ml with priming before the stimulation test. There is evidence that sex steroid priming makes the testing less likely to overdiagnose GH deficiency. However, most pediatric endocrinologists do not use sex steroid priming. As with other aspects of GH testing, the scientific data are not simple and unequivocal; the result is disagreement and controversy.

• **Different methods for measuring GH in blood samples.** Different labs use different methods (called assays) for measuring GH in the blood samples sent them. Not all these methods agree. Some read a little higher, others lower.

• **Day-to-day variability.** Studies have shown that if growth hormone testing was done exactly the same way on the same child on two consecutive days, it was not uncommon for one test to have a peak of less than 10 and the other test to have a peak above 10. This again suggests there is nothing magical about a child having a growth hormone test result less than 10. For children with severe deficiency (say, a peak growth hormone of below 3), the results tend to be more reproducible.

• **Overweight children.** If children are growing well but happen to be overweight, their growth hormone levels will often be low. So if we find low GH levels in a short, overweight child, it's hard to know whether those values come from true deficiency or just increased body weight.

The Tendency to Overdiagnosis

A number of studies suggest that current testing methods tend to overdiagnose GH deficiency. This tendency may have an underlying psychological cause. Many parents want to be able to do something that will help their child grow taller. Physicians often have a natural tendency to want to help. After all, a family comes to a doctor with a concern. It is sometimes hard to send the family away without "fixing the problem." Making the diagnosis of growth hormone deficiency gives the physician something to offer the family.

Growth hormone can be prescribed even if the child does not receive a diagnosis of growth hormone deficiency. If other causes of short stature have been excluded and the child is short enough, he or she might receive growth hormone under new Food and Drug Administration prescribing guidelines for idiopathic short stature (discussed further in chapter 12). In fact, the doctor could prescribe growth hormone even if the child does not meet any FDA indication guidelines. In the United States, a doctor can legally prescribe medications outside FDA indications (within certain bounds). However, insurance companies are much more likely to pay for the treatment if the child carries a diagnosis of growth hormone deficiency. Therefore, practically speaking, treatment may not be financially feasible if the child has not been given such a diagnosis.

In our view, however, overdiagnosis has important drawbacks. First, an incorrect diagnosis of growth hormone deficiency will lead to the wrong follow-up tests. An MRI of the pituitary may be done when the doctor should be on the alert for a completely different disorder causing growth problems. Second, an incorrect diagnosis of growth hormone deficiency tells a child and his or her parents that the child has a defect in the pituitary gland. The child now incorrectly believes that he or she has an illness. Third, an incorrect diagnosis deprives families of their right to make a fully informed decision about growth hormone therapy. If the doctor tells the family that the child is not making a normal amount of growth hormone, then the family will almost certainly want to give the child back the missing hormone. They will feel that they are restoring the child to normal health. However, if the doctor tells the family that their short child does not have a deficiency, the family will understand that therapy is adding extra growth hormone to the normal levels already produced by the child's pituitary gland. In this situation, some families will still favor treatment, while others won't. We think it's important to try as best we can, given the tests available, to make an accurate diagnosis to allow parents to make a fully informed decision.

Some parents who are sure that they want growth hormone treatment for their child will welcome a diagnosis of deficiency, whether it's accurate or not, because it will increase the likelihood that insurance will cover the cost of treatment. Many parents, however, want an accurate diagnosis. What can parents do to prevent their child from being incorrectly diagnosed as having GH deficiency? It is sometimes helpful to let the pediatric endocrinologist know your concerns during your first visit. Hopefully, this will lead to an open discussion about how these difficult issues affect your child's individual situation. If you are concerned, in some cases you may wish to obtain a second opinion from another pediatric endocrinologist.

With All These Problems, Why Do GH Testing at All?

Because there are so many problems associated with growth hormone stimulation testing, some pediatric endocrinologists have suggested that we abandon it altogether and rely instead on growth patterns and the IGF-I and IGFBP-3 tests. However, GH stimulation tests do have some value. A very low test (such as less than 3 ng/ml) does really suggest a deficiency, while a normal peak level suggests that the child is not deficient. Values in between, however, are hard to interpret.

Our practice is to order these tests mainly in children who have clinical evidence of growth hormone deficiency, based on the severity of the short stature, the pattern of growth, the medical history, the physical exam, the bone age X-ray, and the laboratory studies. Testing children who appear to be "short normal" and do not have clinical evidence of growth hormone deficiency increases the number of incorrect diagnoses.

SPONTANEOUS GROWTH HORMONE TESTING

Are there any alternatives to GH stimulation tests? A different approach is called spontaneous GH testing. In this test, the child is not given any medication. Instead, blood is drawn through an IV frequently (typically every 20 minutes) for hours (usually overnight). Each sample is tested for GH, and the results can be used to see how much GH the child is actually making on his or her own—"spontaneously." A paper published in 1984 suggested that spontaneous testing identified some children with GH deficiency who had been missed by stimulation tests. The authors proposed a new term to describe this phenomenon: growth hormone neurosecretory dysfunction. The intended meaning of this term is that these children might be able to produce an adequate amount of GH after taking a potent medication in a GH stimulation test, but they're not making enough GH on their own because the neural pathways that lead to GH secretion are not functioning normally. However, this study had some weaknesses, and subsequent studies that corrected the shortcomings did not confirm the findings. These more recent studies suggest that spontaneous GH testing is not usually worthwhile except perhaps in certain special circumstances, such as in a child who has had radiation to the brain.

Over the years, the number of medical centers doing spontaneous GH testing has declined, not only because it is inconvenient to draw blood every 20 to 30 minutes for 12 to 24 hours as well as difficult to interpret the result, but also because insurance companies simply stopped accepting this test as proof of GH deficiency.

DIAGNOSIS OF GH DEFICIENCY: OUR OVERALL ASSESSMENT

There is no "gold standard" test that tells us for sure which child has growth hormone deficiency and which child doesn't. It is generally believed that GH deficiency, like most other conditions in medicine, is not all or nothing, and there is a spectrum of deficiency from mild to moderate to severe. In cases of severe growth hormone deficiency, our tests are usually adequate, but in milder cases we are left with uncertainty.

BRAIN MRI FOR CHILDREN WITH GROWTH HORMONE DEFICIENCY

When the diagnosis of GH deficiency has been made, it is important for the doctor to think about the underlying cause (see table 9). Usually, the best way to find an underlying cause is an MRI of the brain with a special focus on the pituitary gland. As mentioned earlier, the most urgent situation is in the child who appears to have acquired, not congenital, growth hormone deficiency, where we are particularly worried about the possibility of a tumor or other potentially progressive problem in or near the pituitary gland. In this situation, a brain and pituitary MRI is usually done as soon as the diagnosis of growth hormone deficiency is made. An MRI is especially important for children who have poor growth plus some other sign of a tumor, such as visual disturbance or headaches that are becoming more severe and more frequent.

In children with severe congenital growth hormone deficiency, an MRI is also often performed, because it sometimes turns up an abnormality in the size or configuration of the pituitary gland or other associated abnormalities in the brain structure. In children with possible mild GH deficiency who are otherwise healthy, an MRI is unlikely to show an abnormality.

KEY POINTS TO KEEP IN MIND

GH deficiency can occur by itself or in combination with other pituitary hormone deficiencies. It can be caused by a wide variety of problems involving the pituitary gland or brain. These problems can be congenital or acquired. The diagnosis of growth hormone deficiency is most often made by doing stimulation tests. While the tests we order usually provide a clear result in children with severe deficiency, these tests have many problems, and, as currently performed, probably tend to overdiagnose growth hormone deficiency. When clear-cut deficiency is identified, the doctor will usually order an MRI of the brain and pituitary to look for the cause.

CHAPTER 11

Treatment of Short Stature

We have reviewed the causes of short stature, the psychological impact of being short, and the problems with diagnosis of growth hormone deficiency. We are now ready to discuss the treatment of short stature. It is a subject of considerable controversy, which will be explored further in chapter 12. In that chapter, we will state our opinion that the great majority of short children do not need treatment, which should be considered only in certain specific situations. However, before we can explain our viewpoint, we need to discuss the available treatments, how effective they are, and what drawbacks they have. Only then can we rationally consider which short children might benefit from treatment. The main subject of this chapter will be the use of growth hormone for treating short stature, but we will also cover the use of androgens (male hormones) and medications to delay puberty.

A BRIEF HISTORY OF GROWTH
HORMONE THERAPY

The era of human GH therapy began in the late 1950s, when growth hormone, obtained from human pituitary glands collected at autopsy, was injected into a small number of very short children suspected of having growth hormone deficiency. The results were very impressive even though the amount of growth hormone available to treat these children was very small by today's standards. In 1960, a group of physicians in the United States, recognizing the importance of this new form of treatment and wishing to avoid a black market in the scarce growth hormone, established an organization called the National Pituitary Agency (NPA), whose mission was to collect as many pituitary glands as possible, purify the growth hormone they contained, and make it available to patients who needed it the most. They enlisted the cooperation of a group of pathologists who performed autopsies—a difficult task because it took extra time to remove the pituitary gland, about the size of a pea, from the base of the brain. The participating pathologists would freeze the glands and then ship them in batches to the NPA for processing.

The dose of growth hormone used at that time was less than half that which most US patients are started on now. It was recognized that higher doses were more effective, but there wasn't enough growth hormone to go around. To treat as many children as possible, physicians were provided enough growth hormone to treat most patients for only eight months out of the year. Despite these obstacles, the shortest and most severely deficient patients usually did get the growth hormone they needed and in most cases responded very well.

The year 1985 was momentous in the annals of growth hormone therapy. In the spring of that year, four cases of a rare neurological disease called Creutzfeldt-Jakob disease (CJD for short) were identified in young adults who had received pituitary growth hormone 10 to 20 years earlier. The early symptoms of this incurable illness were loss of balance and dementia, but in some cases the diagnosis was not made until an autopsy was done on the brain. It was recognized that this illness, which is similar to other degenerative brain diseases including mad cow disease, can be transmitted through eating or being injected with infected nervous tissue. A few of the pituitary glands used to produce batches of pituitary growth hormone must have come from people who had CJD. Officials of the National Institutes of Health, the Food and Drug Administration, and the Centers for Disease Control reacted swiftly. Distribution of pituitary growth hormone was halted in the spring of 1985, and the endocrine community braced for a large number of deaths of their former patients, since each batch of growth hormone included material from thousands of pituitary glands and was distributed to perhaps hundreds of patients. Attempts were made to contact every single pituitary growth hormone recipient. It was a bleak time for everyone involved.

There were, fortunately, fewer cases of CJD than we had

feared. As of 2003, 26 cases of CJD had been found in the United States among nearly 8,000 people who had received pituitary growth hormone. Similar cases also occurred in other countries.

In 1985, a positive and exciting event also occurred. Genentech, one of the first biotech companies, announced that it was ready to market the first biosynthetic growth hormone (produced in genetically engineered bacteria). The work that resulted in this scientific breakthrough went back to the 1970s, when scientists first developed methods to isolate and clone DNA. DNA, the genetic material in each cell, encodes the "instructions" for making all of our proteins, including human growth hormone. Genentech scientists successfully inserted the gene for growth hormone into a common intestinal bacteria, called *E. coli*, which could be grown in large quantities. Methods had to be developed to "fool" the bacteria into producing large quantities of GH, and then to purify it by removing all the other proteins in the bacterial soup. Finally, in the fall of 1981, after testing it in adults for safety, approval was obtained from the FDA to begin tests with biosynthetic growth hormone in children with proven GH deficiency. At this time, I (Paul Kaplowitz) was doing my fellowship training in pediatric endocrinology at the University of North Carolina at Chapel Hill, which was one of about 10 sites testing the new growth hormone. I gave the first two patients their first growth hormone injections, an event that was captured in photographs shown the next day on the front page of the *Durham Morning Herald*.

No one was surprised that biosynthetic growth hormone, which was virtually identical to pituitary growth hormone, worked quite well in children with GH deficiency; in fact, it seemed to work even better, because the dose recommended by Genentech was more than twice that which had been used with pituitary growth hormone. It took another four years, however, to collect the safety and effectiveness data needed to obtain FDA approval for the treatment. It finally became available to patients in the fall of 1985, only a few months after pituitary growth hormone had been withdrawn from use.

CONDITIONS TREATED WITH GROWTH HORMONE

Growth hormone is, of course, used to treat GH deficiency. For the child who is truly growth hormone deficient, GH treatment is replacing a missing hormone, and the treatment tends to reverse many of the abnormalities found in this condition, including the short stature. There is general consensus in the pediatric endocrinology community that this treatment is appropriate in that the benefits outweigh the risks.

However, the treatment is also used in children who are short but not growth hormone deficient. In these other conditions, we are not replacing a missing hormone. We are giving extra growth hormone, trying to raise levels to compensate for some other growth problem that we may or may not understand. Growth hormone will accelerate growth in children with short stature due to many conditions. However, there is considerable controversy about the medical and ethical issues. For some of these conditions, there is sufficient evidence regarding safety and efficacy that the FDA has approved the use of growth hormone. Still, even in these conditions—listed below—growth hormone therapy is just an option; the risks and benefits must be carefully weighed in each individual child.

Turner Syndrome

Turner syndrome, discussed in chapter 7, is a condition in which girls are missing part or all of one X chromosome. These girls are not growth hormone deficient, but they are quite short. In 1996, Turner syndrome was approved by the FDA as an indication for growth hormone treatment, because studies had shown that girls with this condition could grow an extra 3 to 5 inches above what would have been predicted at the start of treatment. This could make the difference, for example, between a girl ending up at least 5 feet tall, instead of 4 feet, 9 inches. The earlier the condition is diagnosed, the earlier growth hormone can be started, and the greater the potential increase in height. The initial growth response in such girls is not as great as that seen in growth hormone deficiency, but the growth rate will generally improve. The recommended dose is about 25 percent higher for girls with Turner syndrome than for children with growth hormone deficiency. Figure 11 shows the growth chart of one of our patients who was started on growth hormone at the age of five, when her adult height was predicted to be only 4 feet, 6 inches. By age 16, when the treatment was stopped, she had reached about 4 feet, 11 inches, an increase of about 5 inches. Not all girls with Turner syndrome respond this well, but we wanted to illustrate how growth hormone, if started early enough and given long enough, can substantially increase height.

Prader-Willi Syndrome

Another condition for which growth hormone has recently been approved is Prader-Willi syndrome. There is some evidence that these children do, in fact, have partial growth hormone deficiency, but the issue is complicated. In these children, growth hormone treatment does increase the growth rate, but perhaps the more important effects are reduced body fat, increased muscle mass, and improved ability to participate in physical activities. However, GH is by no means a miracle cure, and these children continue to have major medical problems. In addition, several deaths have been reported in such children during therapy due to obstruction of the breathing passages. At this point, it is not certain whether growth hormone caused these deaths, but parents considering treatment should carefully discuss the risks and potential benefits with their pediatric endocrinologist.

Children Born Small for Gestational Age
Who Do Not Catch Up on Their Own

In 2001, the FDA approved GH for short children who were born small for gestational age. To qualify—as you

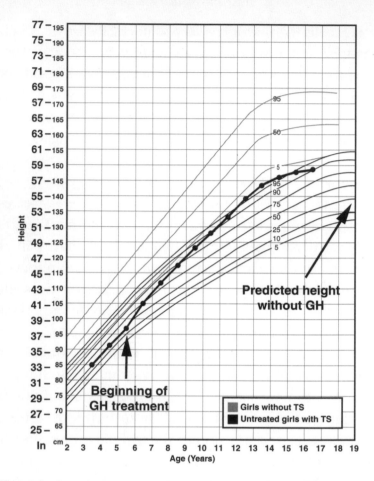

Figure 11. Growth chart of a child with Turner syndrome (TS). The chart shows the normal range for girls with the syndrome and those without. The individual girl with Turner syndrome plotted here was initially on the 25th percentile for Turner syndrome. Modified from a growth chart provided by the Turner Syndrome Society. Used with permission.

might expect—a child must have been born small for gestational age. For a child who was born at full term, this is defined as a birth weight of 5 pounds, 8 ounces (2,500 grams), or less, or a birth length of 18 inches or less. Charts are available showing the birth weights for infants born prematurely below which a child is considered to have been small for gestational age. Since many such children experience catch-up growth in the first two years of life, the child must still be below the normal range for height at two years of age or later. The recommended dose of growth hormone is about 60 percent greater than that typically used for children with growth hormone deficiency, as studies have shown that there is faster catch-up growth—at least in the first two years—with the higher doses, and that the incidence of side effects does not appear to be greater than with the standard doses.

Chronic Renal Failure

Growth hormone is also approved for children with short stature due to chronic kidney failure. Poor growth in these children has many causes but is not due to lack of growth hormone. However, giving growth hormone to such children causes a significant increase in their growth rate, at least in the short term.

Idiopathic Short Stature

In 2003, the FDA approved the use of growth hormone for children with idiopathic short stature who meet certain criteria. This treatment is so controversial that we will spend much of chapter 12 discussing it in more detail.

Conditions Not Approved by the FDA for Growth Hormone Treatment

For many of the causes of short stature listed in chapter 7, growth hormone treatment has not been approved by the FDA. Doctors can still legally prescribe growth hormone for these conditions. In most cases, however, we have only limited data about the safety and efficacy of growth hormone. For some, we have evidence that it accelerates growth in the short term but no proof that it increases the child's eventual adult height. In some of these conditions, there are special concerns about certain risks, such as the risk of cancer. Because safety and efficacy have been less well studied in these disorders, doctors are generally more reluctant to prescribe growth hormone outside FDA indications. Also, insurance companies are much less likely to pay for the treatment.

GH THERAPY AND QUALITY OF LIFE

Many parents and physicians assume that growth hormone treatment will not just increase the growth rate and adult height of the child, but also consequently make the child happier and better adjusted. In this discussion, we will put aside the effects of GH on children with severe deficiency and focus instead on the much larger group of children who have idiopathic short stature. However, the same issues that we will consider may also apply to other non-growth-hormone-deficient children, such as those born small for gestational age or even those with Turner syndrome.

Does growth hormone treatment result in important psychological benefits? The results of studies are conflicting, in part, because some had important design flaws. In one of the early studies looking at this question, researchers tested 109 children with GH deficiency and 86 children with idiopathic short stature during three years of growth hormone treatment. Compared with children of normal height, both groups of short children appeared to have more behavioral problems prior to treatment and these problems appeared to decrease during treatment, with the effect being greater in the GH-deficient group than the idiopathic short stature group. However, this study did not include a group of children who remained untreated, for comparison with the treated group, and thus it is hard to know if the improvement was actually caused by the growth hormone. In another study that was better designed, 36 children with idiopathic short stature were randomly assigned to GH treatment or no treatment. After two years, compared with the untreated group, the group receiving growth hormone showed a significantly greater growth rate, but neither the parents nor the children reported any improvement in the children's self-esteem or health-related quality of life—a measure that combines physical, psychological, and social well-being. This study, then, would suggest that growth hormone does not improve quality of life. However, the duration of treatment in this study was fairly brief—only two years—and the number of children studied was small. In yet another study, a group of children with idiopathic short stature was treated with growth hormone for four years and compared with a control group receiving placebo injections. The data suggested a possible trend toward improvement in problem behaviors, as measured by questionnaires completed by the parents. This result was not clear-cut, however, and no effects were observed on other psychological measures.

In our opinion, these and other related studies do not provide a conclusive answer as to whether growth hormone treatment has a significant impact on psychological function or quality of life. Part of the problem is that psychological well-being is much harder to measure than height. We can measure height with a great deal of accuracy, but psychological measures are not nearly that precise. Furthermore, psychological well-being and quality of life may be influenced by many factors besides height, such as health, family relationships, friendships, and school performance. It may be very difficult to discern the effect of height on quality of life when so many other variables play a role. And finally, to look at the larger picture, do we need to prove that growth hormone treatment improves overall quality of life in order to justify it? Or is it enough that some people with extreme short stature are distressed by their physical difference and want their height to be closer to normal?

COMMON QUESTIONS ABOUT GROWTH HORMONE TREATMENT

When a growth specialist recommends a course of growth hormone therapy for a short child, many questions are likely to occur to parents. In the next pages, we'll try to answer these questions, summarizing both published studies and our own collective 40 years of experience treating short children.

Why Does Growth Hormone Need to Be Given by Injection?

Growth hormone cannot be given orally because it is a protein, and therefore would be digested in the stomach by the same enzymes that help digest meat and milk proteins. Some hormones, including thyroid hormone, hydrocortisone, and estrogen, can be taken by mouth, but they are small molecules unaffected by digestive enzymes. Not so with GH, which is therefore administered by an injection just under the skin (subcutaneously) using very small needles, similar to those used to inject insulin. Currently, most of the companies that produce growth hormone package it in sealed cartridges, which are inserted into a special injection device. A special type of needle called a pen needle—even thinner than the needle on a typical insulin syringe—is then attached to the cartridge and the correct dose is dialed in, rather than drawn up into a syringe. The discomfort associated with pen needle injections is even less than with insulin syringes, but some children may still be very anxious about starting injections. Many parents are concerned about how well their children will tolerate the injections and uncertain about whether they themselves will be able to administer them. However, we find that most children and parents cope well with the injections, and children are often surprised at how little they actually hurt compared with other shots they may have received. There is currently one preparation of growth hormone on the market that is actually sprayed though the skin without needles. This way of giving growth hormone is not painless, but it may be preferred by some children who have a fear of needles.

Research is currently under way to determine whether growth hormone can be given by inhalation into the lungs. The hormone may be absorbed into the lungs and then into the bloodstream. If this approach proves safe and effective, children may be able to receive growth hormone using an inhaler similar to those used to treat asthma.

How Much Does Growth Hormone Cost?

The price of growth hormone has not increased since its biosynthetic form was first marketed in 1985, but it is quite expensive. The larger the child, the greater the dose needed, and therefore the greater the annual cost. As a rule of thumb, the cost is about $10,000 per year for a small child (one who weighs about 30 pounds), $20,000 per year for a larger child (about 60 pounds), and $30,000 or more for a child of 90 pounds or more. About two-thirds of the cost is what the pharmaceutical company charges for it; the other third covers the fees of the pharmacy or home health care agency that processes the order, bills the insurance company and family, and ships the drug to the family.

How Is the Proper Dose Determined?

In the United States, the dose of growth hormone is usually calculated based on the child's weight. Thus we usually talk about the dose in milligrams (one thousandth of a gram, abbreviated mg) per kilogram (abbreviated kg, equal to 2.2 pounds) of body weight per week. Before 1985, when the only growth hormone available was that extracted in limited quantities from pituitary glands, the usual weekly dose was 0.12 mg per kg of body weight per week, divided into three doses. It was recognized, however, that this was not the optimal amount of growth hormone for stimulating growth, and when biosynthetic growth hormone became available, Genentech recommended a starting dose of 0.3 mg per kg per week—more than twice as much. So, for example, a 20-kg (44-pound) child might be given 1.0 mg six times a week, which totals 6 mg per week (0.3 mg per kg per week x 20 kg). Studies showed that this higher dose was somewhat more effective, but not twice as effective. When Eli Lilly and Company, another pharmaceutical company, began to market its version of growth hormone in 1987, it recommended (based on its own studies) a dose of 0.18 mg per kg per week, but most physicians tended to use the higher dose suggested by Genentech. However, for children with the most severe deficiency of growth hormone, the smaller doses often work quite well.

During treatment, different physicians use different strategies to adjust the dose of growth hormone. Some recalculate the dose of growth hormone at every visit to adjust for weight gain; in the example given above, then, if the 20-kg child's weight increases to 22 kg after six months of therapy, they would increase the dose to 1.1 mg six times a week, to maintain the dose at 0.3 mg per kg per week. Other physicians reason that the key determinant of how much growth hormone to use is how well the child is growing. Thus, in the example above, they might keep the dose at 1.0 mg six times a week at the second visit if the child is growing very well (as is usually the case during the first year or two of treatment), and not increase the dose for several visits as long as the child continues to grow at a rapid rate. When the growth slows at a future visit, they might then increase the dosage to 0.3 mg per kg per week.

In the past few years, another approach to adjusting the dose of growth hormone has been proposed. It is argued that we should base our dose adjustments, at least in part, on the blood level of the growth factor IGF-I, trying to keep it in the middle of the normal range for the child's age. This suggestion is partly based on studies showing a possible link between IGF-I levels in blood and the risk of certain cancers in normal adults. It is also possible that use of IGF-I may help adjust for an individual's sensitivity to growth hormone and may decrease the risk of side effects.

The approach to dosing is evolving as more data become available. For now, in most children, we start treatment with the standard recommended dose based on the child's diagnosis and body weight. However, if the child is growing very well, we may not increase the dose for body weight in future visits; occasionally, we may even decrease the dose. We measure IGF-I and usually decrease the growth hormone dose if the IGF-I level is on the high side, but would not increase the dose if the IGF-I is on the low side but growth is good. If your child is on growth hormone, the pediatric endocrinologist should assess the child's individual situation and then discuss any dosage adjustment with you.

How Often Is Growth Hormone Administered?

During the early days of growth hormone therapy, it was standard to give injections only three times a week. Then several studies revealed that, particularly during the first year, administering growth hormone daily was somewhat more effective than giving it three times a week, even if the same total weekly dose of growth hormone was used; today, daily growth hormone has become standard. Many pediatric endocrinologists prescribe growth hormone to be given six days a week instead of daily. We find that some children like being able to select one day a week when they do not need an injection. The same total weekly dose of growth hormone is generally used in both six- and seven-day-a-week regimens, and any difference in effectiveness is probably very small.

Investigators have also looked at whether the time of day when growth hormone is given makes a difference. In normal children, the biggest surge of growth hormone is released after the onset of sleep, and so it might be advantageous to give injections at night rather than in the morning to more closely mimic what occurs naturally. However, studies have not found any difference in the growth response to morning versus evening injections. Many patients do take their growth hormone at night, primarily because that time of day is less rushed than the morning in most homes.

When Should Growth Hormone Be Started?

In children with severe GH deficiency, treatment is usually started as soon as the diagnosis is established. In children who were born small for gestational age, GH is generally not started until sometime after age 2 to see whether the child will catch up on his or her own.

In idiopathic short stature, the age chosen to start treatment depends on various factors. For an adolescent with an advanced bone age, there is little remaining growth potential and therefore less opportunity for GH to have much effect. Starting at a young age allows for a longer treatment period and therefore probably will produce a greater effect on adult height. However, starting early in childhood and treating for many years also increases the cost and might increase the unknown risks of treatment.

Furthermore, very young children (3 years of age or less) may be less cooperative with the injections.

How Do We Know the Hormone Is Working?

Prior to treatment, a typical child with short stature grows at a rate of 1½ to 2 inches per year; children with severe growth hormone deficiency may be growing more slowly (1 to 1½ inches per year). The children who grow the slowest prior to treatment tend to be the ones who have the greatest increase in growth rate when started on growth hormone. If the growth hormone is working, we will see an increase in the child's growth rate (inches of growth per year) by the time of the first visit after starting, typically three to four months later. It is important for parents to be aware that the best response to growth hormone usually occurs during the first four to eight months of therapy.

Children who respond well to growth hormone often see a doubling of their growth rate during the first year of treatment, so that if they were previously growing at 1½ inches per year, we would hope that, after starting treatment, they would grow at least 3 inches per year, at least initially. The child with severe growth hormone deficiency frequently grows 4 inches or more during his or her first year of treatment (see figure 12). For children who respond well to GH, the growth chart usually shows that the height is catching up to the normal percentile curves. A child whose growth rate increases by less than 1 inch per year during treatment is often considered a nonresponder.

If the response is minimal during the first year of treatment (assuming the measurements are accurate), the chances are not good that it will improve in the future. If the increase in growth is well below what the doctor was expecting, and there is no obvious explanation (for instance, the child was ill for a substantial part of the interval, or many injections were missed), you and your child's endocrinologist may have to reconsider whether treatment is beneficial and sometimes even reconsider the diagnosis. If a child is in puberty, it is more difficult to assess the response because puberty itself can cause a large increase in the rate of growth. In any case, your pediatric endocrinologist should guide you through this process.

Regular follow-up visits are needed to be sure that growth hormone is actually doing its job and is not having any side effects. The interval selected by the endocrinologist for follow-up is generally about every four to six months, but some endocrinologists will want to see the patient more frequently, especially at the beginning of treatment.

The response to growth hormone, while usually good initially, wanes after the first year of therapy. If a child with a pretreatment growth rate of 1½ inches per year increases to 3 inches in the first year but then grows at the slower rate of 2½ inches per year during the second year, this second-year growth rate is still well above baseline. We say that the child is still having catch-up growth. In children who respond well to growth hormone, catch-up growth may continue for two to four years. During this time, the child will often move on the growth chart from well below the 3rd percentile to a point closer to or above the 3rd percentile. At some point, however, many children will stop experiencing catch-up growth and start tracking along one of the normal percentile channels, at least until the age of puberty (see figure 12). Short children who reach the normal range during their first few years of treatment will usually be able to remain within the normal range with further treatment and usually achieve a normal adult height.

When Is Growth Hormone Treatment Stopped?

As mentioned earlier, growth hormone treatment may sometimes be stopped if a child does not respond well to it or has some side effect. If the response is satisfactory, treatment is usually continued until the child has achieved a reasonable height or is almost finished growing. Most specialists will stop treatment around the time that the rate of growth decreases to less than 1 inch per year, especially if the child is late in puberty and the bone age has reached 13 to 14 years in girls (96 to 98 percent of adult height) or 15 to 17 years in boys (97 to 99 percent of adult height). Some children with moderate to severe growth hormone deficiency may benefit from continued treatment in adulthood, even though growth is complete. In such adults, there is evidence that growth hormone can help to maintain good muscle mass, increase the amount of calcium in bones, decrease body fat, and have other

CDC Growth Charts: United States

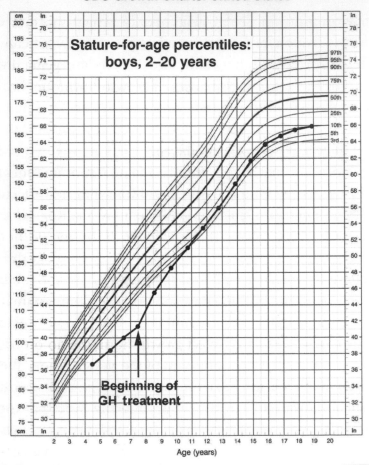

Stature-for-age percentiles: boys, 2–20 years

97th
95th
90th
75th
50th
25th
10th
5th
3rd

Beginning of GH treatment

Age (years)

Modified from NCHS growth charts:
Published May 30, 2000.
SOURCE: Developed by the National Center for Health Statistics in collaboration with
the National Center for Chronic Disease Prevention and Health Promotion (2000).

CDC
SAFER·HEALTHIER·PEOPLE™

Figure 12. Growth chart of a boy with severe, congenital growth hormone deficiency treated with GH. After treatment, beginning at seven years of age, he began to grow very quickly, causing his height to catch up into the normal range. Over the following years, his growth rate on treatment slowed down so that his height tracked almost parallel to the normal percentile curves. Not all children, particularly those with less-clear-cut growth hormone deficiency, respond this well to treatment.

benefits. However, most diagnoses of growth hormone deficiency should be reconfirmed before treatment is continued or resumed in adulthood. Adults are generally treated with much lower doses of growth hormone than are children and adolescents.

How Safe Is Growth Hormone Therapy?

One of the most frequently asked and important questions about growth hormone therapy is what side effects can be anticipated and how serious they are. The good news is that most children on growth hormone do not have any noticeable, significant side effects. On the other hand, serious side effects do occasionally occur, and there is also the possibility that problems may become apparent in the future that are not recognized today.

The needles used to inject growth hormone do on occasion puncture one of the tiny blood vessels under the skin, so a child being treated with growth hormone may at any time have one or more bruises at the sites of recent injections. These occasional bruises generally clear up after a week or two. Because growth hormone given as a medication has the same chemical composition as that made by the body, it is uncommon for the body to develop either a local reaction or an allergy to it.

Still, treatment often provides more growth hormone than is normally made in the body. Perhaps as a result, treatment is associated with certain uncommon but important side effects. Some, but not all, of these effects are reversible if the growth hormone is stopped.

One such uncommon problem is an increase in the pressure of the fluid that surrounds the brain. This condition is called pseudotumor cerebri, or benign intracranial hypertension. The typical symptoms include headaches, impaired vision, and/or vomiting. This side effect usually occurs within the first months of treatment. The condition will usually resolve if the growth hormone is stopped. After the problem resolves, if the child has a strong indication for GH treatment, the injections may be restarted at a lower dose, and the problem sometimes does not recur.

Growth hormone treatment can decrease the body's sensitivity to insulin, the hormone that regulates blood sugar levels. The body will respond by producing more insulin, thus preventing a significant increase in blood sugar. However, there is some evidence that a rare child may be pushed over into diabetes. The diabetes in question is not primarily the very severe type in which the insulin-producing cells of the pancreas are destroyed by an autoimmune disease (called childhood-onset); rather, it is the adult-onset type of diabetes (which can also occur in children). This type of diabetes may not be quite as severe as the childhood-onset form and can sometimes be treated with oral medication, but it is still a serious disease. The association between growth hormone treatment and diabetes isn't certain, and if it is real, diabetes is still a rare complication. Nevertheless, to be careful, we try to stay alert to the small possibility of a child developing diabetes after starting growth hormone. The typical symptoms of diabetes are increased drinking and urination. In addition, pediatric endocrinologists will sometimes check blood glucose levels at office visits in children on growth hormone, particularly if they think the risk of diabetes is increased.

Another uncommon possible side effect of growth hormone therapy is slipped capital femoral epiphysis. This condition involves the ball-shaped upper end of the femur (thighbone), which forms part of the hip joint. In slipped capital femoral epiphysis, the end of the femur slips relative to the rest of the femur. Parents and doctors of patients on growth hormone should be on the lookout for hip, leg, or even knee pain. It seems to be more common in older children; the average age of diagnosis is more than 14 years. If suspected, it can be diagnosed by taking X-rays of the hips. The majority of cases require surgery, in which an orthopedic surgeon can stabilize the femur by inserting pins.

The risk of growth hormone that parents tend to worry about most is cancer. The first report that growth hormone treatment might increase cancer risk was published in 1988 based on a Japanese study. It was found that a number of GH recipients in Japan developed leukemia (a cancer of the white blood cells) at what was thought to be a higher-than-expected rate. Since then, however, the incidence of leukemia in children treated with growth hormone has been studied in the United States and other countries. The studies suggest that growth hormone does not increase the risk of leukemia in children who have no other risk factors for this type of cancer. In children who do already have an increased risk of leukemia—for example, those who have received treatment for a prior tumor—it is more difficult to establish or exclude an effect of growth hormone.

A study published in 2002 described a group of 1,848 patients who had received pituitary growth hormone as children. In these patients, the risks of mortality from cancer overall, colorectal cancer, and Hodgkin's disease (a cancer involving lymph nodes) appeared to be significantly increased compared with the general population. However, the actual number of patients with these disorders was small (10 deaths from malignancy, two cases of colorectal cancer, and two cases of Hodgkin's disease), and therefore there is uncertainty about the association between growth hormone and cancer risk. Still, there is a plausible scientific basis for this finding, since growth hormone causes levels of IGF-I to increase. IGF-I can make healthy cells divide more rapidly, and cancers may be more likely to occur when certain cells are growing and dividing more rapidly. In addition, studies suggest that patients with very high levels of growth hormone due to pituitary tumors may have an increased risk for colon polyps and colon cancer. Furthermore, some studies have shown a statistical association between IGF-I levels in normal adults and the risk of certain cancers. This possible increased risk is one of the reasons some specialists now recommend monitoring IGF-I levels during GH therapy, since in theory higher IGF-I might increase the cancer risk. Although there have been many studies in this area, none has been absolutely definitive, and we still do not know with certainty whether growth hormone treatment increases the risk of cancer and, if so, by how much.

For children whose growth hormone deficiency has occurred as a result of a brain tumor, there is the additional worry that treatment might stimulate growth of any remaining tumor cells and therefore increase the risk of recurrence. Although brain tumor recurrence is not rare, no studies to date have found a definite increase in the risk of tumor recurrence specifically related to GH therapy. The existing studies are far from definitive, though, and therefore uncertainty exists in this situation as well. It is common practice to wait at least a year after diagnosis and treatment of a brain tumor before considering growth hormone treatment.

Scoliosis (curvature of the spine) is a fairly common problem in children and adolescents. There is some evidence that scoliosis may occur or worsen when growth is accelerated by growth hormone treatment. Therefore, children should be examined for scoliosis before and during GH therapy.

We have not tried to discuss every complication that might be associated with growth hormone therapy but have instead focused on those considered the most important and/or most likely to be associated with treatment. In addition, we should remember that we may not yet know all the complications of GH therapy. For example, there could be complications that will not become apparent until large numbers of patients treated with growth hormone in childhood reach middle or old age. Of course, this same consideration applies to most medications that we give children.

In addition to the health risks, there is a possible psychological risk to giving growth hormone. It has been suggested that giving growth hormone to a child without GH deficiency might send a message that short stature represents a handicap or an illness.

The bottom line, in our opinion, is that most children who receive growth hormone treatment do not have any detectable, important side effects, but there are some uncommon complications and some additional risks that might be associated with treatment. Therefore, we have to balance the possible risks against the possible benefits. There is a consensus in the pediatric endocrinology community that, in children with severe growth hormone deficiency, the benefits outweigh the risks. At the other end of the spectrum, in healthy children who are simply in the lower part of the normal range and likely to end up somewhere within the normal range, almost everyone would agree that the risks outweigh the benefits. The difficulty is deciding where to draw the line between these two extremes. This issue is discussed more fully in chapter 12.

TESTOSTERONE AND ANABOLIC STEROIDS

In certain situations, the use of male hormones to stimulate growth is as effective as growth hormone and far less expensive. A vial of testosterone for injection, which is more than enough for this form of treatment, costs only $60 to $80. Many of the short boys we see are 14 or older and have constitutional delay of growth, which we discussed in chapter 7. Their height is often below the 3rd percentile, but because they have not yet started their pubertal growth spurt, they still have good growth potential; based on their delayed bone age, they often have a predicted height in the range of 5 feet, 5 inches, to 5 feet, 9 inches, the lower half of the normal range. If left alone, these boys will likely enter puberty and start to grow rapidly in the next year or two. The problem is that some are distressed because they feel different from their peers who have already started puberty. Not only are they smaller, but also they lack the body hair and genital changes associated with puberty and often have a more childish appearance, a higher voice, and less muscle than their peers. In boys who are distressed by these physical differences, some physicians perform growth hormone testing—and because of problems with the tests discussed earlier, these tests may erroneously indicate GH deficiency in a healthy late-maturing boy. If these boys are started on growth hormone treatment, they probably will grow faster initially than they would otherwise. However, once puberty starts, the effect of growth hormone becomes hard to distinguish from the effect of puberty. In this situation, the use of growth hormone is usually unnecessary, and the cost and risks, in our opinion, usually outweigh the benefit.

Another approach in this situation is to offer short boys

who are late in entering puberty a short series (usually about four) of monthly injections of testosterone dissolved in oil (to prolong its effectiveness). The usual dose is 50 to 100 mg per monthly injection, which is about one-eighth to one-quarter of what is used for replacement therapy in a man who is unable to produce testosterone. It is usually given by a nurse in the office of the primary care doctor who referred the patient. Testosterone typically causes a rapid increase in growth hormone secretion, IGF-I production, and growth. One of us (Paul Kaplowitz) has published results indicating that a boy who may have grown only 1½ to 2 inches in the previous year will grow an average of 1½ inches during the four months of testosterone injections. Also, the boy will generally develop other physical changes typical of puberty. In most cases, the boy's own reproductive system will become activated after the injections are completed and puberty will continue to progress. This treatment will not make a child taller than he would have been if he had been left alone, but it will get him to a normal height sooner and help normalize his puberty, both of which can be important to a teenage boy. A typical growth curve for a boy treated with testosterone at age 14½ is shown in figure 13.

Parents often ask why giving testosterone, which results in the child's growth ending sooner, does not make the child *shorter* than he would have been. Fortunately, the available evidence suggests that on average, this treatment, if given to boys age 14 or older, has little if any effect on adult height. One of us (Paul Kaplowitz) has by now given

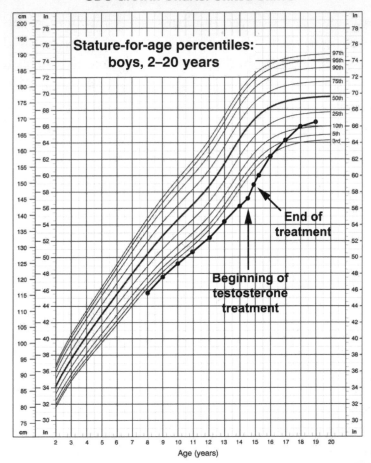

CDC Growth Charts: United States

Stature-for-age percentiles:
boys, 2–20 years

End of treatment

Beginning of testosterone treatment

Modified from NCHS growth charts:
Published May 30, 2000.
SOURCE: Developed by the National Center for Health Statistics in collaboration with
the National Center for Chronic Disease Prevention and Health Promotion (2000).

Figure 13. Growth chart of a boy with constitutional delay of growth treated with low-dose testosterone injections. At 14½ years old, he was short and had no signs of puberty. He received four monthly injections of low-dose testosterone, which caused an increase in his growth rate and early signs of puberty. At that time, he started to go into true puberty and continued to grow well and catch up to the normal range. Not all children respond this well to treatment.

testosterone to close to 100 boys with constitutional delayed puberty, and in nearly every case, growth improved impressively and continued to be good after the injections were stopped. The boys are generally pleased with both their rapid growth and the growth in size of their genitals and the amount of pubic hair. Perhaps because the hormone provided is the same one normally made during puberty, is given at a modest dose, and is usually given for only four to six months, the risks of testosterone appear low. However, testosterone treatment should be considered only in certain patients, mainly those who have reached age 14, have not started puberty (or have only just started), have an adult height prediction within the normal range, and are distressed by their delayed puberty or growth.

Parents may be wondering at this point why we do not give testosterone by pill, since it is not digested in the stomach the way growth hormone is. There *is* a pill form of testosterone, but it has been found to cause liver problems in some patients, so we tend to avoid it. If doctors do want to give a male hormone in pill form, they generally use one of the synthetic male hormones (also known as anabolic steroids) in small doses for a period of 6 to 12 months. The one that has been most studied is oxandrolone (brand name Anavar). When used in appropriate doses for this purpose, it appears to have a low incidence of side effects. One theoretical advantage that it has over testosterone is that it is less likely to speed up bone maturation, because unlike testosterone, it cannot be converted into estrogen.

DELAYING PUBERTY AS A WAY OF IMPROVING GROWTH

Puberty can be shut down by medications called gonadotropin-releasing hormone (GnRH) agonists (or analogs), thus allowing more time for growth and possibly increasing adult height. These medications are long-acting, modified forms of a hormone made in the hypothalamus that triggers the pituitary gland to produce gonadotropin hormones, which in turn stimulate the testes or ovaries to produce testosterone and estrogen at the time of puberty. The most commonly used medication in this class is leuprolide (brand name, Lupron Depot). Lupron, as it is commonly called, is given as a monthly injection, and it effectively blocks the production of gonadotropins and sex steroids (androgens and estrogens) from the testes or ovaries. For years, we have used this medication to treat children with precocious puberty (puberty that starts at an abnormally early age). Blocking production of sex hormones slows the rapid increase in bone maturation and allows these children to grow for a longer period of time before their growth plates close. It therefore helps them to reach an adult height closer to their genetic potential, while without treatment, some of these children would end up quite short.

Lupron and similar drugs have also been used to treat children who have puberty at a normal age but are very short. This treatment tends to slow the advancement in bone maturation and delay the closure of the growth plates, again allowing these children to grow for a longer period of time and end up slightly taller than they would have been otherwise. A recent study showed that pubertal delay for an average of 3½ years resulted in a modest increase in adult height—on average 1½ to 2 inches. One major drawback to this approach, however, is that a child started on medication at age 12 would not have further progression through puberty for several years, and during that time, he or she would actually grow less than if allowed to go though puberty normally. These effects during adolescence might increase the child's distress. The payback is that such children will continue to grow until they are 17 or 18, after other children are done. Another potential problem is that the treatment causes a decrease in bone density that is in some ways similar to what occurs in women after menopause. It is not known whether the bone density will fully recover after the treatment is stopped. If it doesn't, these children might be at increased risk for osteoporosis. As with any medication, there is also the risk of unknown side effects. While Lupron is not as expensive as growth hormone, it is hardly cheap at approximately $10,000 per year. The FDA has not approved this treatment, and we think that it should not be used routinely in children with short stature. We would only consider it in a child who is beginning puberty and has an extremely short predicted adult height, when the physician, parents, and child all feel that the modest benefit justifies the major drawbacks mentioned above.

A combination of Lupron and growth hormone treatment has been tried in very short children who are starting puberty and have a very low predicted height. Some studies have suggested an increase of 3 to 4 inches in adult height if this combination is used for at least three years, but the studies are not conclusive, and the combined therapy entails all the risks and costs of both medications. This combined treatment is not approved by the FDA and, as far as we know, is not often prescribed.

Recently, a different class of medications, aromatase inhibitors, has been tried experimentally to treat short stature in boys. Aromatase inhibitors, which are given orally, block the conversion of androgens to estrogens. This type of medication is approved by the FDA for use in women with breast cancer; it's effective because it deprives the cancer cells of estrogen. Some preliminary studies show that an aromatase inhibitor called letrozole (Femara) can also, by blocking estrogen production in teenage boys, cause bone maturation to slow and therefore allow more time for growth. Because androgen production is not blocked, the boys would continue to have the usual physical changes of puberty. Although the approach sounds promising, at the time we are writing this book, there remains some uncertainty about the effectiveness of the treatment and more uncertainty about its safety. The safety of letrozole has been studied in many women with breast cancer in whom the side effects include a probable increased tendency toward osteoporosis. However, the safety of letrozole has not been well studied in boys, and there is reason to think that blocking estrogen production in an adolescent boy might have additional, important side effects that might not be present in older women (whose estrogen production is already low because they are past menopause). Letrozole is not likely to be a safe and effective treatment for adolescent girls with short stature because blocking estrogen production in the more active ovaries would probably entail additional problems. The Food and Drug Administration has not approved letrozole or any other aromatase inhibitor for the treatment of short stature.

KEY POINTS TO KEEP IN MIND

Growth hormone is currently used to treat children with GH deficiency and certain other causes of short stature. Even if the short stature is not due to growth hormone deficiency, growth hormone treatment will usually accelerate growth, at least initially. Most children who receive growth hormone treatment have no detectable, important side effects, but there are some uncommon complications and some possible risks. Growth hormone also has other drawbacks, including its cost and the discomfort of injections. Some boys who are short because of delayed maturation are treated with androgens, which can accelerate growth and help initiate puberty. In children who are very short but do not have delayed puberty, a medication can be given to postpone puberty; this allows more time for growth and may increase adult height. However, this treatment has its own important drawbacks. Because all these treatments have disadvantages, the risks and benefits must be carefully weighed in each situation.

CHAPTER 12

The Growth Hormone Controversy

In the previous chapter, we discussed growth hormone treatment in general, including its risks and benefits. As we indicated, growth hormone is now used to treat not just children with growth hormone deficiency but also some other children who are very short for other reasons. We will now focus on the most controversial part of the growth hormone story: its use in short children with no identifiable cause for their short stature, usually referred to as idiopathic short stature, which was just recently approved by the FDA. The controversy involves the ethical issues of treating short but otherwise healthy children, and also the financial issues of using this expensive treatment in a society in which the cost of health care is increasing rapidly and in which limited resources are sometimes inadequate even for standard medical care. Some insurance companies are refusing to pay for this controversial use of growth hormone. Although we focus this discussion on idiopathic short stature, many of the same issues apply to other non-growth-hormone-deficient conditions such as being born small for gestational age and Turner syndrome.

COMMON QUESTIONS ABOUT GH TREATMENT FOR IDIOPATHIC SHORT STATURE

How Effective Is It?

There is solid scientific evidence that growth hormone does increase height in children with idiopathic short stature. During the first year of treatment, the average rate of growth typically increases from 1½ to 2 inches per year to about 3 to 3½ inches per year—a fairly good response in most cases. As noted in chapter 11, the response generally falls off in the second year, but many children are still growing better than before treatment. Until recently, however, it was not known whether children receiving growth hormone treatment would actually end up taller as adults. It was considered possible that they would grow faster but stop growing sooner and thus end up at the same adult height.

There are now several studies in which children with idiopathic short stature have been treated with growth hormone long enough to determine the effect on adult height. Although none of the studies is perfect, they strongly suggest that growth hormone treatment can increase the adult height of children with idiopathic short stature. The exact amount of the average increase is less clear. In one recently published study, growth hormone appeared to produce an average increase in adult height of only 1½ inches. However, the dose of growth hormone was fairly low (0.24 mg per kg per week, rather than the more typical 0.3 mg per kg per week), the treatment was given only three times per week (rather than the usual six or seven times per week), and the treatment was started fairly late in childhood (about 12 years of age) so that the children received on average about four years of treatment. Other studies suggest that the effect of growth hormone on adult height would be greater if it were given in a higher dose and given daily. How much greater effect? It's hard to know. An educated guess is that a typical child might gain something like 2 to 3 inches, but again, this is just a guess based on indirect evidence. Also, the effect is likely to vary considerably in different children. It also probably would depend on the age when the treatment was started and the number of years that the child was treated. Some research- ers are trying to find better ways to predict which children will show the greatest increase in adult height.

How Safe Is It?

As far as we can tell, the safety profile for growth hor- mone is similar in children with idiopathic short stature to the safety profile in other conditions such as Turner syndrome or GH deficiency. Thus, there are some known side effects, some side effects that might be related to treat- ment, and the possibility of unknown risks, especially long-term risks. These are reviewed in chapter 11. Still, as with other conditions treated with growth hormone, the large majority of children have no evident, significant side effects.

Which Children with Idiopathic Short Stature Are Included in the FDA-Approved Guidelines?

The FDA-approved guidelines do not include all children with idiopathic short stature. For example, they don't include the very common situation in which a child is at the 5th or even the 3rd percentile. This child is likely to be the shortest kid in the classroom, but he or she is not short enough to meet the FDA guidelines. The FDA approval specifies that children must be less than the 1st percentile (or, to be exact, 2.25 standard deviations below the mean, which is the 1.2 percentile). Table 10 shows the height at different ages corresponding to this percentile. This means that the majority of children (about four out of five) who are below the 5th percentile are not eligible for growth hormone under these guidelines. The FDA-approved indication also specifies that GH should be used only in those children who would not be expected to achieve a normal height without treatment. Thus, growth hormone would not be indicated for a boy with constitutional growth delay who was below the 1st percentile but had a bone age delayed enough that he would likely achieve an adult height in the normal range (5 feet, 4 inches, or greater for boys).

Table 10. 1st Percentile Heights

Height in Inches Corresponding to the 1st Percentile

Age in Years	Boys	Girls
4	36½	36
5	38¾	38½
6	41	41
7	43¼	43¼
8	45½	45½
9	47¼	47
10	49	48¾
11	50½	50½
12	52¼	53
13	54½	55¾
14	57¼	57½

Heights corresponding approximately to the 1st percentile (2.25 standard deviations below the mean) for children age 4 through 14 years. Under the FDA-approved guidelines for idiopathic short stature, growth hormone is indicated only for children who are as short as or shorter than the 1st percentile (approximately). Each height in the table represents the approximate cutoff value for a child on his or her birthday. For example, 45½ inches is the value for a girl 8 years and 0 months old. The value for a girl 8 years and 6 months old would be approximately halfway between the values for an 8-year-old and a 9-year-old girl. The FDA-approved guidelines also specify other criteria besides the child's current height.

THE CONTROVERSY

The use of growth hormone to treat children with idiopathic short stature is highly controversial. Many arguments have been advanced for and against it. We will list some of the salient ones, on both sides.

Arguments Against Growth Hormone Treatment

- **Idiopathic short stature is a normal variation.** Critics of broadening the indications for growth hormone treatment often view idiopathic short stature as a normal variation. Some kids are tall, some average, some short. These individuals would argue that idiopathic short stature is just the name for children in the lowest part of the range. They are otherwise healthy. Medicine should be concerned with treating disease. Treatment of idiopathic short stature is cosmetic.

- **Short stature does not cause significant disability.** Those opposed to growth hormone treatment cite the evidence, some of which was mentioned in chapter 8, suggesting that short stature is not associated with major psychological problems. Furthermore, there isn't good evidence that growth hormone treatment will improve self-esteem, quality of life, or other psychological outcomes.

- **The risks outweigh the benefits.** There are known side effects of growth hormone therapy and possible unknown risks. We should not expose children to any risk unless there is a compelling need. Being short is not a compelling need.

- **Growth hormone treatment causes inequities.** Allowing wider access to growth hormone for all children who are below the 1st percentile, it has been suggested, will not eliminate the problem of short stature in our society, but will confer an advantage on those short children whose parents are aggressive enough to push for treatment or wealthy enough to pay for it if it isn't covered by insurance.

Children whose parents are either not as aggressive or less wealthy will be left farther behind.

- **Growth hormone treatment is too expensive for our society.** Another key issue is whether wider use of growth hormone, considering its cost, is a good use of health care dollars at a time when the costs of health care and health insurance are skyrocketing. The money might be better spent on prevention and treatment of serious disease. We will explore this issue in more detail later.

Arguments for Growth Hormone Treatment

- **Whether a child is entitled to growth hormone should not depend on the cause of the short stature.** Advocates of growth hormone therapy for idiopathic short stature have posed the following argument. Imagine you have two children, Jill and Jane. Both are the same age and the same height—extremely short. Both have the same predicted height, which is well below the normal range. Jill has growth hormone deficiency (or Turner syndrome), whereas Jane has idiopathic short stature. Both will respond to growth hormone. Why should Jill be entitled to growth hormone treatment and Jane not?

- **Extreme short stature is not normal.** Some growth hormone proponents argue that it is not normal to be extraordinarily short. It is a failure of the bones to grow normally. In idiopathic short stature, we simply do not know the cause of the abnormality. As time goes by, research will continue to identify genetic abnormalities causing the short stature.

- **Some individuals with short stature are distressed by their physical difference.** Although studies have not shown major psychological dysfunction in short stature, that may be an unfair measure. Many factors may influence a person's quality of life and overall psychological status, including health, friendships, family relations, and school or job success. Therefore, it may be hard to detect the influence of any one factor, such as height. Perhaps it is enough that some children with extreme short stature are unhappy about their height. Some short children report that they are bullied, teased, or treated as if they are much younger than they really are. Some short adults also are distressed by the way they are viewed and treated by others. Isn't that enough reason to treat? If a child has a birthmark on the face that he or she finds cosmetically unpleasant, do we deny treatment because there are no studies showing that treatment will increase overall quality of life?

- **Growth hormone testing is inaccurate.** Other proponents of treatment point to the inaccuracy of growth hormone testing in defining who is actually growth hormone deficient and who is not, as we discussed in chapter 10. Why, they ask, should a very short child who happens to pass her testing (with, for example, a peak growth hormone level of 11 ng/ml) be denied growth hormone while another child would be approved for treatment because his peak growth hormone level was 9 ng/ml? If the child with a slightly lower test result was much more likely to respond to GH, this would make sense. However, several studies have shown that children with a peak growth hormone over 10 ng/ml and those with a peak below 10 respond to growth hormone similarly, at least in the short term (except for those with a very low growth hormone response, who may respond better).

• **Some extremely short individuals experience physical barriers.** Individuals who are extraordinarily short may, for example, have trouble driving a car or seeing where they are going in a crowd.

Our Viewpoint

We think that growth hormone treatment is not appropriate for the large majority of children with short stature. The typical child who is at or above the 3rd percentile should, in general, not be treated. In this situation, the disadvantages of treatment, especially the risks and cost, outweigh any benefit that the individual might derive from an increase in height. On the other hand, we do not agree with the absolute approach that growth hormone is never appropriate for idiopathic short stature. We think that growth hormone treatment may be considered in the occasional child who is:

- Unusually short. A child at the 1st percentile, conceivably, but more so the child who is well below the 1st percentile. We are also more likely to consider treatment in a child who is falling farther away from the normal range with time.

- Unlikely to achieve a normal height as an adult. Here we have to rely on predicted heights tempered by clinical judgment.
- Not adjusting well psychologically to his or her physical difference.

This final criterion needs some explanation. Some children seem to adjust well to the fact that they are shorter than their peers. Many short children are popular, excel in academics or in sports, or just have a wonderful positive attitude and do not find their height to be a major problem. In these children, there is less pressure to incur the costs and risks of growth hormone treatment. If we could only purify and bottle this positive attitude, it would be the best treatment for short stature.

However, other children seem quite distressed by their height. They think about it frequently and wish very much to be taller. It is hard to know if their unhappiness is really caused by the short stature or just blamed on the short stature. If they were taller, would they still be unhappy, but about something else? We are not criticizing the child who is distressed by short stature; different children have different personalities. We can admire the short child with an upbeat, can-do attitude, and we can empathize with the child who is troubled. However, in the child who is quite distressed, there is more impetus to consider treatment. Some parents, particularly parents of young kids, may argue that their children may not be distressed now, but will probably be troubled when they are older. Each case must be considered individually. Ideally, the child, the parents, and the growth specialist will together carefully weigh the advantages and disadvantages and come to a consensus about the best course. However, if the decision is made to treat, one additional party has to be convinced—the insurance company.

THE HIGH COST OF GROWTH HORMONE

Many parents are surprised when they learn how much the growth hormone treatment they are considering will cost, even when they are responsible for little to none of the bill. We mentioned in chapter 11 that for most children, the cost of growth hormone falls between $10,000 and $30,000 per year, though it can be even higher in a larger teenage child. And a course of growth hormone is rarely limited to a year; the cost for five years of treatment can easily exceed $100,000.

Many people have a difficult time understanding why this drug (and others) should be so expensive, and they may blame the problem on corporate greed. While it is not our mission to defend drug companies (neither of us owns shares in any companies that market growth hormone), we think this may be an oversimplification. We should point out that years of expensive basic research go into producing any drug. Conducting clinical trials to test for safety and efficacy is extremely costly and can take years. Only about 20 percent of new drugs that reach human trials are eventually approved. Most drugs that go through this long period of development and testing never even make it to market. On average, it costs the pharmaceutical industry almost a billion dollars for each drug that is brought to market. Unless pharmaceutical companies reap a large profit from each "hit," they will stop doing the enormously costly research that will provide all of us with future drugs. Curtailing profits too much might be like killing the proverbial goose that laid the golden egg.

Also, it is worth noting that, despite the high rate of drug price inflation over the last two decades, the wholesale cost of growth hormone has remained flat since it was introduced 20 years ago, and growth hormone is not expensive when compared with other biotechnology drugs. What makes the overall cost so high is that growth hormone is taken not for weeks or months, but in many cases over a period of 5 to 10 years, and each year the dose—and therefore the cost—increases as the child grows.

As more and more companies began to market their own preparation of growth hormone (at this writing, there are six different companies marketing growth hormone in the United States), some people expected that competition would drive the price down, but this has not happened. Perhaps part of the reason might be that pharmaceutical companies suspect that any price cut they make will be matched by other companies; thus it wouldn't increase market share but simply decrease profits. Also, most families pay little if any of the cost of growth hormone; therefore a decline in price would mainly benefit insurance companies, not parents.

Insurance Company Resistance to Paying for
GH for Idiopathic Short Stature

In the United States, insurance companies and Medicaid pay the lion's share of the bill for growth hormone. There are no national consensus guidelines as to who should receive growth hormone, so each company and Medicaid program is free to develop its own. Insurance companies are constantly being asked to cover more and more expensive and high-tech treatments, while trying to rein in costs and keep premium increases at reasonable levels. Although they are not legally bound to cover treatments that have been approved by the FDA as appropriate for a particular situation, they usually do so. Thus, when the FDA approved growth hormone for Turner syndrome, most insurance companies eventually went along; the same thing occurred when the FDA approved GH for children born small for gestational age who had not caught up by two years old.

The response to the FDA approval of growth hormone for idiopathic short stature has been somewhat different, however. Many insurance companies have reviewed their guidelines on whom to cover for growth hormone therapy and decided that they do not consider growth hormone for idiopathic short stature medically necessary. If insurance companies revised their guidelines so that even children who passed the testing were eligible for treatment, the number of children under their plan who would qualify for growth hormone might increase significantly. To agree to cover a course of growth hormone for 1 percent of the children in a plan at an eventual cost of more than $100,000 per child is viewed by some health insurance companies as an unacceptable threat to the bottom line. Presumably, this increased expense would eventually be passed on by raising insurance premiums. Some of this extra cost would be paid directly by families and the rest by employers, who, in turn, might pass on increased costs to employees by switching to plans with higher annual employee premiums, higher co-pays, and higher deductibles. Our point here is that the hard-line response of many insurance companies is understandable: Increasing access to growth hormone for short children ends up costing everyone within the health plan more money. On the other hand, if your own child is extremely short and you feel that the benefits outweigh the risks of growth hormone in your situation, you may be very frustrated to learn that your insurance company refuses to pay.

So is there a reasonable middle ground? The current system relies almost completely on growth hormone stimulation tests, which do a poor job of predicting who will actually benefit from treatment. What would happen if we simply did away with growth hormone testing and treated children on the basis of how short they are?

There is one large-scale experience with such an approach to treating short stature, from Australia. There, health care costs are covered by the government rather than private insurance companies, and the use of growth hormone is regulated by an expert national committee. In 1988, this committee decided that growth hormone should be available to any child below the 3rd percentile in height whose growth rate over the previous year was somewhat low. After seeing how many children qualified for treatment with growth hormone, and noting that the cost to the government was well above estimates, the height cutoff was changed in 1993 to the 1st percentile (approximately the same as the idiopathic short stature cutoff approved by the US FDA). Since then, growth hormone usage has been stable, and the cost has been manageable. The Australians believe that their current policy makes for a judicious and effective use of growth hormone in their country. This approach, however, is not likely to be adopted in the United States. Here, there is no government-sanctioned expert committee, and the decision about payment for treatment is in the hands not of the federal government but hundreds of different insurance companies (and, in the case of children covered by Medicaid, 50 different state Medicaid programs).

Inequities in the System

For the near future, insurance companies will probably continue to scrutinize requests for growth hormone treatment in an attempt to hold down costs. And perhaps that scrutiny will have a positive consequence: It may prevent some mildly short children from being treated inappropriately. Unfortunately, the process by which decisions are made regarding treatment not only varies greatly from one insurance company to another, but also ends up covering growth hormone for many who don't need it while denying coverage for some children for whom treatment is reasonable. For example, one child may have constitutional growth delay or mild familial short stature, but he might be approved for growth hormone treatment because, when tested, he happened to have a peak growth hormone level a little less than 10. Another child who might be far shorter relative to her peers might be denied approval by the insurance company because she reached a growth hormone level of 12 during her stimulation testing.

How We Could Improve the System—Our Two Cents

The system might work more equitably if a few changes were made. First, growth hormone deficiency could be defined more strictly, based on the severity of the short stature, the growth pattern, evidence of other pituitary hormone deficiencies, the levels of IGF-I and IGFBP-3, and perhaps more rigorous GH stimulation testing. Second, children with severe (not mild) idiopathic short stature and a predicted height well below normal could be eligible for growth hormone treatment if the family and growth specialist think that the potential benefit to the child is worth the cost and risks. Third, cases in which the decision is not clear-cut could be referred by insurance companies for review by outside physicians with expertise in treating growth disorders. Currently, these cases are generally reviewed by individuals within the health plan with little expertise in this area, and decisions are often based solely on the company's inflexible written guidelines.

KEY POINTS TO KEEP IN MIND

Growth hormone treatment is now approved by the FDA for use in some children who are not GH deficient, including those with idiopathic short stature below the 1st percentile. This indication is controversial, opposed by those who think it is unnecessarily subjecting normal children to a medical treatment and supported by those who think that the cause of short stature should not determine ethically who is treated. We favor an intermediate approach: Growth hormone is inappropriate for the large majority of children with short stature but can be considered in the much less common situation of a child who is extremely short, is unlikely to catch up to the normal range by the time he or she is done growing, and is not adjusting well to the physical difference.

SELECTED REFERENCES

Chapter 3

American Academy of Pediatrics Staff, et al. *American Academy of Pediatrics Guide to Your Child's Nutrition: Making Peace at the Table and Building Healthy Eating Habits for Life.* New York: Random House, 1999.

Lifshitz F. 1993. Fear of obesity in childhood. Ann NY Acad Sci 699:230–6.

Northwestern University Web site on nutrition: www.feinberg .northwestern.edu/nutrition/factsheets/protein.html.

Pencharz PB. Body composition and growth. In Walker A, ed. *Nutrition in Pediatrics: Basic Science and Clinical Applications.* Boston: Little, Brown, 1985:77–85.

Sanders TA. 1988. Growth and development of British vegan children. Am J Clin Nutr 48(Suppl 3):822–5.

Silventoinen K. 2003. Determinants of variation in adult body height. J Biosoc Sci 35(2):263–85.

Treasure J, Schmidt U. 2004. Anorexia nervosa. Clin Evid 11:1192–203. Update of: Jun 2003. Clin Evid 9:986–96.

United States Department of Agriculture Web site: www .mypyramid.gov.

Chapter 4

Allen DB. 2004. Systemic effects of inhaled corticosteroids in children. Curr Opin Pediatr 16:440–4.

Larsen PR, Kronenberg HM, Melmed S, Polonsky KS, eds. *Williams Textbook of Endocrinology*, 10th ed. Philadelphia: Saunders, 2003.

Lee PA. 2003. The effects of manipulation of puberty on growth. Horm Res 60(Suppl 1):60–7.

Pedersen S. 2001. Assessing the effect of intranasal steroids on growth. J Allergy Clin Immunol 108(Suppl 1):S40–4.

Van der Eerden BC, Karperien M, Wit JM. 2003. Systemic and local regulation of the growth plate. Endocr Rev 24:782–801.

Wickman S, Sipila I, Ankarberg-Lindgren C, Norjavaara E, Dunkel L. 2001. A specific aromatase inhibitor and potential increase in adult height in boys with delayed puberty: a randomised controlled trial. Lancet 357:1743–8.

Chapter 5

Halac I, Zimmerman D. 2004. Evaluating short stature in children. Pediatr Ann 33:170–6.

Web site to find growth charts: www.cdc.gov/growthcharts. Hyattsville, MD: US Department of Health and Human Services, Centers for Disease Control and Prevention (CDC). National Center for Health Statistics (NCHS). National Health and Nutrition Examination Survey Data.

Chapter 6

Bramswig JH, Fasse M, Holthoff ML, von Lengerke HJ, von Petrykowski W, Schellong G. 1990. Adult height in boys and girls with untreated short stature and constitutional delay of growth and puberty: accuracy of five different methods of height prediction. J Pediatr 117:886–91.

Greulich WW, Pyle SI. *Radiographic Atlas of Skeletal Development of the Hand and Wrist.* Stanford, CA: Stanford University Press, 1959.

Hintz RL. 2001. Final height prediction in constitutional growth delay. J Pediatr Endocr Metab 14:1535–40.

Maes M, Vandeweghe M, Du Caju M, Ernould C, Bourguignon JP, Massa G. 1997. A valuable improvement of adult height prediction methods in short normal children. Horm Res 48:184–90.

Chapter 7

Allen DB, Bielory L, Derendorf H, Dluhy R, Colice GL, Szefler SJ. 2003. Inhaled corticosteroids: past lessons and future issues. J Allergy Clin Immunol 112(Suppl 3):S1–40.

Ashkenazi A. 1989. Occult celiac disease: a common cause of short stature. Growth, Genetics, Hormones 5:1–4.

Cezard JP, Touati G, Alberti C, Hugot JP, Brinon C, Czernichow P. 2002. Growth in paediatric Crohn's disease. Horm Res 58(Suppl 1):11–5.

MTA Cooperative Group. 2004. National Institute of Mental Health Multimodal Treatment Study of ADHD follow-up: changes in effectiveness and growth after the end of treatment. Pediatrics 113:762–9.

Chapter 8

Downie AB, Mulligan J, Stratford RJ, et al. 1997. Are short normal children at a disadvantage? Wessex Growth Study. BMJ 314(7074):97–100.

Harper B. 2000. Beauty, stature, and the labour market: a British cohort study. Oxf Bull Econ Stat 62:771–800.

Meyer-Bahlburg HFL. Short stature: psychological issues. In: Lifshitz F, ed. *Pediatric Endocrinology*, 3rd ed. New York: Marcel Dekker, 1990:173–96.

Ross JL, Sandberg DE, Rose SR, et al. 2004. Psychological adaptation in children with idiopathic short stature treated with growth hormone or placebo. J Clin Endocr Metab 89:4873–8.

Sandberg DE, Brook AE, Campos SP. 1994. Short stature: a psychosocial burden requiring growth hormone therapy? Pediatrics 94:832–40.

Sandberg DE, Bukowski WM, Fung CM, Noll RB. 2004. Height and social adjustment: are extremes a cause for concern and action? Pediatrics 114:744–50.

Stabler B, Siegel PT, Clopper RR, et al. 1998. Behavior change after growth hormone treatment of children with short stature. J Pediatr 133:366–73.

Theunissen NCM, Kamp GA, Koopman HM, et al. 2002. Quality of life and self-esteem in children treated for idiopathic short stature. J Pediatr 140:507–15.

Zimet GD, Cutler M, Liverne M, et al. 1995. Psychological adjustment of children evaluated for short stature: a preliminary report. J Dev Behav Pediatr 16:264–70.

Chapter 10

Gandrud LM, Wilson DM. 2004. Is growth hormone stimulation testing in children still appropriate? Growth Horm IGF Res 14:185–94.

Loche S, Bizzarri C, Maghnie M, Faedda A, Tzialla C, Autelli M, Casini MR, Cappa M. 2002. Results of early reevaluation of growth hormone secretion in short children with apparent growth hormone deficiency. J Pediatr 140:445–9.

Mauras N, Walton P, Nicar M, Welch S, Rogol AD. 2000. Growth hormone stimulation testing in both short and normal statured children: use of an immunofunctional assay. Pediatr Res 48:614–8.

Reiter EO, Morris AH, MacGillivray MH, Weber D. 1988. Variable estimates of serum growth hormone concentrations by different radioassay systems. J Clin Endocr Metab 66:68–71.

Rose SR, Ross JL, Uriarte M, Barnes KM, Cassorla FG, Cutler GB Jr. 1988. The advantage of measuring stimulated as compared with spontaneous growth hormone levels in the diagnosis of growth hormone deficiency. N Engl J Med 319:201–7.

Spiliotis BE, August GP, Hung W, Sonis W, Mendelson W, Bercu BB. 1984. Growth hormone neurosecretory dysfunction. A treatable cause of short stature. JAMA 251:2223–30.

Chapter 11

Cronin MJ. 1997. Pioneering recombinant growth hormone manufacturing: pounds produced per mile of height. J Pediatr 131:S5–7.

Frasier SD. 1997. The not-so-good old days: working with pituitary growth hormone in North America, 1956 to 1985. J Pediatr 131:S1–4.

Kaplowitz P. 1998. Delayed puberty in obese boys: comparison with constitutional delayed puberty and response to testosterone therapy. J Pediatr 133:745–9.

Lee PA, Chernausek SD, Hokken-Koelega ACS, et al. 2003. International Small for Gestational Age Advisory Board Consensus Development Conference Statement: management of short children born small for gestational age. Pediatrics 111:1253–61.

Mills JL, Schonberger LB, Wysowski DK, Brown P, Durako SJ, Cox C, Kong F, Fradkin JE. 2004. Long-term mortality in the United States cohort of pituitary-derived growth hormone recipients. J Pediatr 144:430–6.

Swerdlow AJ, Higgins CD, Adlard P, Preece MA. 2002. Risk of cancer in patients treated with human pituitary growth hormone in the UK, 1959–85: a cohort study. Lancet 360:273–7.

Wilson DM, McCauley E, Brown DR, Dudley R. 1995. Oxandrolone therapy in constitutionally delayed growth and puberty. Bio-Technology General Corporation Cooperative Study Group. Pediatrics 96:1095–100.

Yanovski JA, Rose SR, Municchi G, Pescovitz OH, Hill SC, Cassorla FG, Cutler GB Jr. 2003. Treatment with a luteinizing hormone-releasing hormone agonist in adolescents with short stature. N Engl J Med 348:908–17.

Chapter 12

Allen DB, Fost N. 2004. hGH for short stature: ethical issues raised by expanded access. J Pediatr 144:648–52.

Bell J, Dana K. 1998. Lack of correlation between growth hormone provocative test results and subsequent growth rates during growth hormone therapy. Pediatrics 102:518–20.

Leschek EW, Rose SR, Yanovski JA, et al. 2004. Effect of growth hormone treatment on adult height in peripubertal children with idiopathic short stature: a randomized, double-blind, placebo-controlled trial. J Clin Endocr Metab 89:3140–8.

Werther GA, Wang M, Cowell CT. 2003. An auxology-based growth hormone program: update on the Australian experience. J Pediatr Endocr Metab 16 (Suppl 3):613–8.

Wit JM, Rekers-Mombarg LT, Cutler GB, Crowe B, Beck TJ, Roberts K, Gill A, Chaussain JL, Frisch H, Yturriaga R, Attanasio AF. 2005. Growth hormone (GH) treatment to final height in children with idiopathic short stature: evidence for a dose effect. J Pediatr 146:45–53.

Measuring Your Child's Standing Height

For children at least two years old (preferably three).

Materials
- A carpenter's level
- A steel tape measure
- A pencil
- A room with an uncarpeted floor
- An assistant (especially if the child is young)

Step-by-Step Instructions
1. *Make the measurement in the morning. Believe it or not, height decreases a bit during the day.*

2. *Have your child stand barefoot, or in socks, on an uncarpeted floor. Have him or her stand with the back of the heels, buttocks, shoulders, and the back of the head touching a wall.*

3. *Ask your child to stand up straight and tall. He or she should be stretching a little to stand as tall as possible, but you*

should check to be sure that the heels are still flat on the floor. No tiptoes.

4. Be sure that his or her head is level, not looking up or down.

5. Place a carpenter's level over the top of your child's head. Adjust the level until the bubble shows that it is horizontal. If you don't have a level and can't borrow one, you can use another straight object such as a ruler or a piece of wood, but have your assistant stand back and look to be sure it's as horizontal as possible.

6. Mark the wall where the bottom surface of the level touches the wall.

7. Have your child step away from the wall and then back in place. Follow steps 2 through 6 again. Do it all a third time. The marks should generally be within ¼ inch of each other. If not, do it a couple more times and pick one of the middle marks as the best average.

8. Using a steel tape measure, make a measurement from the floor to the mark on the wall. Just to be sure, measure from the floor to the mark again.

Measuring Your Child's Supine Length

For children less than three years old. *Warning:* Measuring supine length is more difficult than measuring standing height. Even experienced personnel have trouble getting accurate measurements.

Materials
- A rectangular object such as a videotape or a CD case
- A steel tape measure
- A room with thin carpeting
- Two assistants!

Step-by-Step Instructions
1. *Dress your child in thin clothing.*
2. *Lay him or her on a floor with thin carpeting with his or her feet close to a wall.*

3. *If your child is in diapers, unfasten the diaper and extend the front portion so that it is lying flat on the ground. This will allow you to bring the legs completely together. You may want to lay another diaper or cloth loosely over your child to avoid an unexpected shower!*

4. *One assistant should bring the legs together and place the feet flat against the wall.*

5. *Next, straighten out the child's body and hold the head in position—facing straight at the ceiling, not tilted left, right, up, or down.*

6. *Now the other assistant should place the rectangular object so that one side is on the floor and another side is touching the top of your child's head. Be careful not to trap his or her hair between the rectangular object and the floor.*

7. *You can now pick up your child while the second assistant carefully keeps the object in place and the first assistant measures the distance from the object to the wall. Whew!*

8. *Repeat it all over again a couple of times. The measurements should be within about ½ inch of each other. Take an average.*

9. *Try to keep your child entertained during the whole procedure. If he or she becomes upset and starts fighting, you might as well give up and try again some other time.*

Plotting Height and Weight on Growth Charts

Growth charts are printed on the following pages; see figures 14–21. These growth charts are a little harder to use than normal growth charts because they are smaller than usual. Alternatively, you may want to use a copy of your child's growth chart from his or her pediatrician. Or you can print out a growth chart from: www.cdc.gov.

Step-by-Step Instructions

1. *Select the appropriate growth chart. First, there are different charts for boys and girls. Second, there are different charts for supine lengths (measured lying down) in young children (age 0–3 years), and for heights in older children (2–20 years). For a child who is 2–3, you could use either chart, but you should not plot a supine length on a height chart or vice versa. Third, there are charts for height, charts for weight, and charts for both height and weight on the same page (not included in this book).*

2. *Choose which units you will use. For some charts (including the ones in this book), it is easier to plot the height in inches and the weight in pounds. These charts also let you use centimeters (cm) and kilograms (kg), but the lines of the grid are matched to the inches and pounds. For other growth charts, the grid lines are matched to centimeters and kilograms, so it's easier to plot using the metric system. If your growth chart is better set up for centimeters and kilograms, you can convert as follows:*

Take your child's height or length in inches and multiply *by 2.54 to convert it to centimeters. Take your child's weight in pounds and* divide *by 2.2 to convert it to kilograms.*

3. *Calculate your child's age in years and months. For example, if your child will have her sixth birthday one month from now, her current age is 5 years and 11 months.*

4. *For practice, try plotting the correct point for a boy, age 10 years and 6 months, who has a standing height of 54¼ inches. Now compare your result with figure 3 on page 55. If you found an x at the point you marked, you did it correctly.*

5. *Now plot your child's height and weight.*

6. *If math was not your favorite subject in school, have someone else check your work.*

Figure 14. CDC Growth Charts: United States

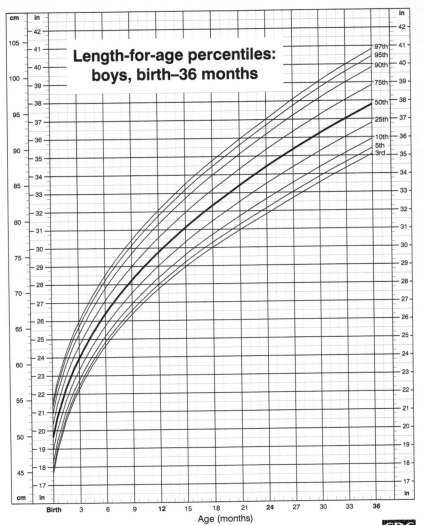

Length-for-age percentiles: boys, birth–36 months

Age (months)

Published May 30, 2000.
SOURCE: Developed by the National Center for Health Statistics in collaboration with
the National Center for Chronic Disease Prevention and Health Promotion (2000).

CDC

SAFER·HEALTHIER·PEOPLE®

Figure 15. CDC Growth Charts: United States

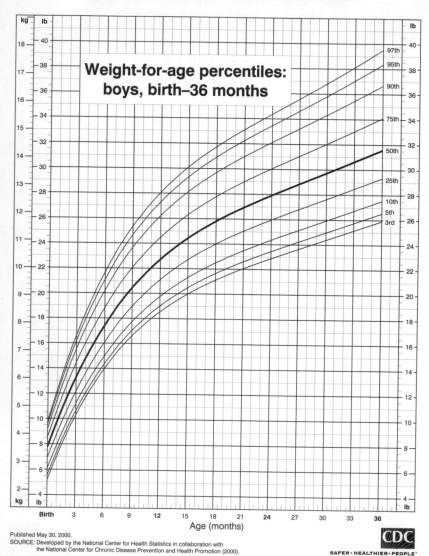

Weight-for-age percentiles: boys, birth–36 months

Published May 30, 2000.
SOURCE: Developed by the National Center for Health Statistics in collaboration with
the National Center for Chronic Disease Prevention and Health Promotion (2000).

CDC
SAFER·HEALTHIER·PEOPLE™

Figure 16. CDC Growth Charts: United States

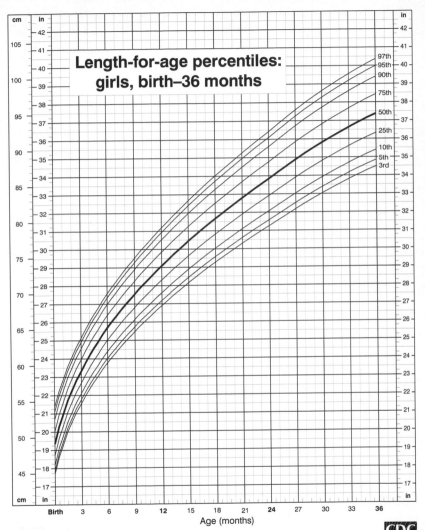

Length-for-age percentiles: girls, birth–36 months

97th
95th
90th
75th
50th
25th
10th
5th
3rd

Age (months)

Birth 3 6 9 12 15 18 21 24 27 30 33 36

Published May 30, 2000.
SOURCE: Developed by the National Center for Health Statistics in collaboration with the National Center for Chronic Disease Prevention and Health Promotion (2000).

CDC
SAFER · HEALTHIER · PEOPLE

225

Figure 17. CDC Growth Charts: United States

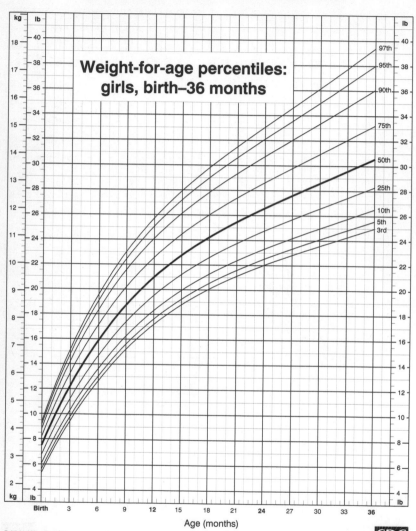

Weight-for-age percentiles: girls, birth–36 months

Published May 30, 2000.
SOURCE: Developed by the National Center for Health Statistics in collaboration with
the National Center for Chronic Disease Prevention and Health Promotion (2000).

CDC
SAFER·HEALTHIER·PEOPLE™

Figure 18. CDC Growth Charts: United States

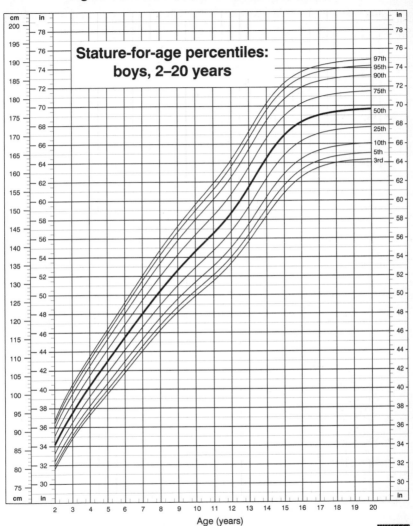

Stature-for-age percentiles:
boys, 2–20 years

Published May 30, 2000.
SOURCE: Developed by the National Center for Health Statistics in collaboration with
the National Center for Chronic Disease Prevention and Health Promotion (2000).

SAFER·HEALTHIER·PEOPLE™

Figure 19. CDC Growth Charts: United States

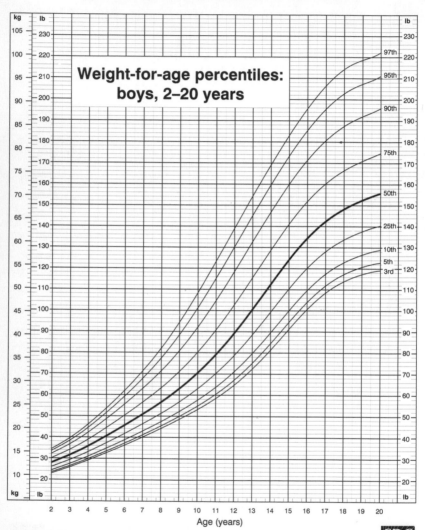

Weight-for-age percentiles: boys, 2–20 years

Published May 30, 2000.
SOURCE: Developed by the National Center for Health Statistics in collaboration with
the National Center for Chronic Disease Prevention and Health Promotion (2000).

SAFER · HEALTHIER · PEOPLE

Figure 20. CDC Growth Charts: United States

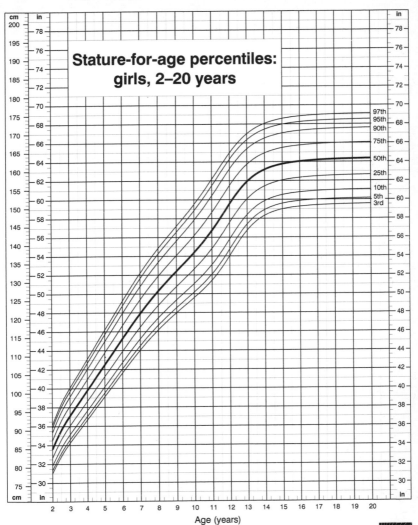

Stature-for-age percentiles: girls, 2–20 years

Published May 30, 2000.
SOURCE: Developed by the National Center for Health Statistics in collaboration with the National Center for Chronic Disease Prevention and Health Promotion (2000).

CDC
SAFER · HEALTHIER · PEOPLE

229

Figure 21. CDC Growth Charts: United States

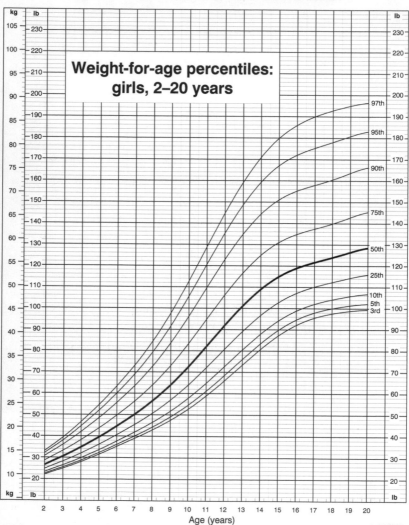

Weight-for-age percentiles: girls, 2–20 years

Published May 30, 2000.
SOURCE: Developed by the National Center for Health Statistics in collaboration with
the National Center for Chronic Disease Prevention and Health Promotion (2000).

INDEX

ABOUT THE AUTHORS

Dr. Paul Kaplowitz is a pediatric endocrinologist with 23 years of experience in treating children with growth disorders. He did his pediatric residency training and pediatric endocrinology fellowship at the University of North Carolina and for 21 years was on the faculty of the Virginia Commonwealth University School of Medicine. In August 2003, he took the position as chief of endocrinology at the Children's National Medical Center in Washington, DC. He has published more than 40 articles and book chapters, mostly in the area of growth and puberty, and in February 2004, Ballantine published his first book, *Early Puberty in Girls: The Essential Guide to Coping with This Common Problem.*

Dr. Jeffrey Baron is a pediatric endocrinologist with 19 years of experience evaluating and treating children with growth disorders and performing scientific research in this field. He completed a residency in pediatrics at Yale and then did a fellowship in pediatric endocrinology at the National Institutes of Health (NIH) in Bethesda, Maryland. He has remained at the NIH and is currently chief of the Section on Growth and Development. He is board-certified in general pediatrics and in pediatric endocrinology. He has published more than 50 scientific papers related to this field. Dr. Baron participated in the authorship in a personal capacity and not as a representative of the NIH or the federal government.